A WOMAN'S
BOOK
OF HERBS

Elisabeth Brooke qualified as a Medical Herbalist with the National Institute of Medical Herbalists in 1980 and opened and runs a training clinic for herbal students in London. She also has a private practice in London and teaches and lectures worldwide.

For more information and contact details, please visit www.elisabethbrooke.com

A WOMAN'S BOOK OF HERBS

Elisabeth Brooke

First published in 1992 by The Women's Press Ltd.

This edition published 2018 by

Aeon Books Ltd
12 New College Parade
Finchley Road
London NW3 5EP

British Library Cataloguing in Publication Data

A C.I.P. for this book is available from the British Library

ISBN-13: 978-1-91159-722-3

www.aeonbooks.co.uk

TO MY MOTHER

The author would like to thank the following:

Starhawk for an extract from *The Spiral Dance: A Rebirth of the Ancient Religion of the Great Goddess: Rituals, Invocations, Exercises, Magic*, published by Harper & Row, San Francisco, 1989.

Marian Woodman for an extract from *The Owl Was A Baker's Daughter: Obesity, Anorexia Nervosa and the Repressed Feminine*, published by Inner City Books, Toronto, 1980.

Mary Daly for an extract from *Websters' First New Intergalactic Wickedary of the English Language*, in cahoots with Jane Caputi, published by Beacon Press, Boston, 1987, and The Women's Press, London, 1988.

CONTENTS

ACKNOWLEDGEMENTS

Writing this book has shown me clearly how little I could do without the support and encouragement of friends and colleagues. The idea came from a plant: thank you lobelia. Fiona Fredenberg said that if I didn't write the book, she would. I did it Fiona! Susan Marionchild taught me psychic skills which led to my esoteric work with plants. To all the women who participated in my esoteric herb workshops, who helped me to develop my theories and put them to the test, and my clients who tried out the remedies and taught me so much.

To Maggie Hyde, the Company of Astrologers, who taught me medical astrology, supervised my case work for several years and giggled with me in Latin classes. To Geoffrey Cornelius, also from the Company of Astrologers, who taught me horary astrology and a respect for the past. To Graeme Tobyn who taught me Latin and gave me important clues on the research. To Nina Nissen who read and reread the book and was midwife to the writer inside me, and without whose encouragement the book would not have been written. To Mary Swale, colleague and dear friend, whose exoteric and esoteric support was always with me. To Delphine Sayer who typed out the manuscript and Helen Stapleton who painstakingly went through the book checking all the facts. To the staff of the Psychosynthesis and Education Trust, especially Diana Whitmore and Judith Firman, who lovingly encouraged me.

To Maxine Holden who encouraged me in my struggle to get the book published and for giving me loving support during the process. To Mary Clemmey who guided me through the new world of publishing and lent me her home to finish the book. To Ros de Lanerolle, who had faith in the book and began its journey into publishing. For Loulou Brown whose meticulous editing has made this a far better book and the whole process almost painless. And for the women at The Women's Press, Katherine Bright-Holmes and Kathy Gale who saw the book through its final stages. And most importantly, to the wonderful inspired women in my life for their cups of tea, hot meals and their love. Thank you all!

Tree calendar

from *The White Goddess* by Robert Graves, pp. 165–204

The tree calendar was believed to be a relic of druidism, orally transmitted. It was also used for divination. Each letter was named after a tree or shrub.

From the *Song of Amergin*, said to have been chanted by the chief bard of the Milesian invaders as he set foot on Irish soil (1268 BC) (see Graves, pp. 205–6)

Dec 24–Jan 20 Birch	B	Beth	I am a stag of seven tines
Jan 21–Feb 17 Rowan	L	Luis	I am a wide flood on a plain
Feb 18–Mar 17 Ash	N	Nion	I am a wind on the deep waters
Mar 18–Apr 14 Alder	F	Fearn	I am a shining tear of the sun
Apr 15–May 12 Willow	S	Saille	I am a hawk on a cliff
May 13–Jun 9 Hawthorn	H	Utah	I am fair among flowers
Jun 10–Jul 7 Oak	D	Duir	I am god who sets the head afire with smoke
Jul 8–Aug 4 Holly	T	Tinne	I am a battle waging spear
Aug 5–Sep 1 Hazel	C	Coll	I am a salmon in the pool
Sep 2–Sep 29 Vine	M	Muin	I am a hill of poetry
Sep 30–Oct 27 Ivy	G	Gort	I am a ruthless boar
Oct 28–Nov 24 Reed	NG	Ngetal	I am a threatening noise
Nov 25–Dec 22 Elder	R	Ruis	I am a wave of the sea

The letters add up to 13 which is the number of full moons in a year and a number sacred to witches.

PART 1

INTRODUCTION

This book is intended to be a celebration of healing plants and of women healers. I hope it is both poetic and practical. It can be read as a story of European plant life and as the collective memory of European people that has built up over the centuries. It can also be read as a mystical journey.

The book can be used by those who practise witchcraft and spellcraft for correspondences, planetary or wicca, or as a practical guide to the use of herbs to heal mind, body and spirit. Plant life is vital for our survival on this planet. We need plants for the oxygen we breathe, as well as for food, shelter, clothing, and even for the pages of this book. Yet despite our great dependence on plants, we know very little about them, apart from how they work physically.

In the 1930s Dr Bach, a homeopath, did some pioneering work on the more subtle characteristics of plants, and his discoveries formed the basis of thirty-eight remedies, using plant essences, for the treatment of varying emotional states.[1] With this book I hope to take his work a stage further and add a flavour of my own.

In the world today the notion of plants as teachers has become alien, but people in ancient times knew that certain plants had magical properties and would, for example, plant borage in a garden where courage was needed, or put a bay tree outside their houses to protect the occupants from burglary. The nature of a plant was known to a great many people in many countries and cultures, an indication that the plants had an internal wisdom or meaning of their own

1

which, if enquired into in the right spirit, would reveal itself.

I came to write this book through a number of routes. First, there were the women in my family, my mother and grandmother, both of whom had a great love of plants and whose houses and gardens were always overflowing with cut flowers, seedlings and blossoming flowerbeds. My first memories are of collecting fallen rose petals from my grandmother's rose garden and making my version of *pot pourri*, quite unaware of what I was doing. Years later I discovered that roses are ruled by Venus in Libra, both of which feature strongly in my astrological natal chart. Even as a child I had an intuitive knowledge of what was good for me.

As an adult, I found myself wanting both to work with people and to be with plants. I studied to be a herbalist, but after four years of ploughing through acres of text books I had hardly seen a plant. After graduation I realised I would have to look further for the knowledge I sought. I studied in more esoteric fields: wicca, astrology, tarot, healing. I developed psychic skills and began to work intuitively with plants, and to my delight discovered there were vast areas of knowledge to be found within each plant. In sharing these skills with other women, it became clear that there was a common source of knowledge emerging from the plants. The women, of whom there are now too many to mention by name, left these workshops feeling they had gained an intimate knowledge of the plants they had worked with, and they become empowered and inspired. Most of us women never forgot the way we had learned; we had transcended the dull process of learning by rote and instead learned through experience. This gave us a real understanding of the healing potential of plants, which previously had been limited to using familiar herbs for first-aid purposes. Sometimes the messages received from plants were urgent and specific. For one of our first meetings we arranged to meet at Samhain (31 October), which is the time when the veils between the worlds – that which separate the world of the living from the world of the dead – are thinner than usual. For that reason I decided to work with magical herbs – datura and skullcap – to see what would happen.

I knew that it was important that this information should be disseminated and that I should try to write some of it down for a wider audience. This was several years ago; unfortunately my phlegmatic temperament put the idea on the backburner until the loud knocking of my conscience was so insistent that I could no longer ignore it.

The writing of this book has taken me to places I would never have imagined. I have learned another language, discovered a whole branch of astrology. With the discovery of the decumbiture method – using astrology for diagnostic purposes – I was able to uncover, piece by piece, the European traditions of herbal medicine which instinctively I knew had existed but which no one seemed to know about. By chance I came upon a group of astrologers who have kept alive these traditions, and under the watchful eye of their members I was able, laboriously, to refine and develop my skill until I could use it in my everyday practice. This in turn lead me to read Culpeper in the original, and one summer I ploughed my way through all his extant works.[2] From these sources I was able to piece together an understanding of the European tradition of herbal medicine.

The principles of European medical astrology, vital to the tradition of herbal medicine, are briefly outlined below.

There are four humours: choleric, phlegmatic, sanguine and melancholic. These are connected to the four elements: fire, water, air and earth. The four humours describe four types in physical, emotional and mental terms. No one can be described as a pure type; we are mostly a mixture of two or sometimes three humours, with one predominating. The herbs, acting as they do through the planetary qualities of hot, cold, moist and dry, balance imbalances of the humours. Thus if a person has too much fire, herbs can cool the fire, using cold, moist remedies. Or they can work to balance out the element fire with hot and dry herbs, thus normalising the choleric humour. Long-term treatments tend to be of the latter kind. Treatment of like with like is called treatment by sympathy, while treatment with the opposite is called treatment by antipathy. Herbs under one planet sometimes seem to have the qualities of another, which is somewhat confusing. For example, the herbs of Venus are mainly hot and dry when one would expect them to be cold and moist like Venus. Similarly, many of the herbs of Mercury, which one would expect to be cold and dry are in fact hot and dry. Why is this? Going back to the two methods of treatment, it can be seen that the majority of the herbs of Venus and Mercury work by antipathy in the sense that they counter the cold illnesses which affect the uterus and the nervous system.

Expressing the energy of fire, the choleric woman is enthusiastic, energetic, intuitive and passionate. Choleric women are initiators, performers, visionaries. Fiery types find the ordinary, mundane world a puzzle and a bore. Often accused of being self-centred and dramatic, more than any other type they tend to mythologise life, fighting causes, acting out life's dramas, pursuing spiritual and philosophical goals. Impetuous and enthusiastic, they have a tendency to ride roughshod over those who are more cautious and thoughtful, dismissing their doubts, contemptuous of their fears, only to find their lack of foresight has once again got them into hot water. Known for their bad temper and impatience, the choleric woman often finds herself in conflict with society, tilting at windmills, challenging the status quo. Women in particular are not encouraged to be independent, assertive, extravert. For all its brashness, fire is easily extinguished, especially by water or earth. Fiery people have to learn to temper their great energy and excitement and become more sensitive and responsive to those around them.

Water is flowing, adaptable, powerful and deep. Phlegmatic people feel. Their emotional life is paramount. Often they surround themselves with a family or clan for the feeling of security and connectedness this gives. Sensitive and empathetic to others, they sometimes lose a sense of who they are or feel invaded or taken over by others. Often very psychic, phlegmatics make good listeners and are to be found in the healing professions. Because of their great sensitivity they are fearful and timid, lacking the courage to assert themselves and always tending to put others first. Easily disorientated, the phlegmatic has to learn to be less empathetic and more direct about her needs and wants. For this reason, phlegmatics are sometimes accused of being manipulating; they find it hard to confront and make demands. Their emotionality and emphasis on relationships are devalued in our society. Phlegmatics tend to be carers, mothers, those who are less concerned with their own desires than with the needs of the underprivileged and those who suffer.

The sanguine woman is concerned with ideas and communication, connecting people, places and concepts. The sanguine type fits best into our culture with its emphasis on the rational, the lightweight, speed and optimism. Airy types usually have an impressive list of friends, even though these friendships may seem superficial to a phlegmatic or melancholic. Moving rapidly through people, situations, relationships and physical space, their energy is legendary. Often accused of being distant and at times cold, the airy type dislikes, and is often deeply threatened by, emotional displays. Airy types like things to be logical, predictable, but emotions are seldom expressed in this way. Sanguine types often run from involvement or deal with their relationships by having several lovers at the same time, coolly able to lie to or deceive their partners. They are more interested in ideal relationships than in the nitty gritty of emotional involvement. Positive, friendly and open, airy people love groups, gatherings, anything social, especially if it has a good cause or altruistic purpose. The lesson for airy people is to learn to connect on a deeper level with people.

Pessimism is the predominant emotion of the melancholic type. She will take things carefully, step by step, unable to take the choleric risks of fire or hope for the best like the sanguine woman. The melancholic earthy type has an important role to play, her pessimism helps to counter the volatility of fire and air, to give them reasonable boundaries, to structure their ideas and put in the groundwork needed for any scheme to take off. Melancholics are found leaf-leting, on phone lines, writing pamphlets, negotiation wage deals, on committees. Melancholics do the duller, less glamorous routine work that their fiery and airy sisters have no time to concentrate on. This can cause resentment, and melancholics harbour slights long and hard. The positive attribute of memory can be detrimentally used to brood on the wrongs they think others have done to them, which is a form of self-imposed mental torture. Like a dog with a bone, they can gnaw on a chance remark or imagined insult and worry enough to make themselves ill, getting more and more depressed and resentful. There is a lot of fear in the melancholic but it is a different kind of fear to that of the phlegmatic. It is more a fear of ridicule, of being wrong or foolish. So they will hold themselves in, bound in Saturn's straight-jacket, lest they make the wrong move. Melancholy is a very English humour – the stiff upper lip; not reacting; very correct; with social nuances outsiders are baffled by, such as dishonesty and pretending to like someone and be interest in them, but privately scorning them. Yet the melancholic often has a very fine mind. The correct use of the mind is the lesson here; to use great mental faculties constructively, to use organisational skills and logic to 'hold' the more mutable humours. Analytical psychotherapy is ideal for melancholics, as this discipline provides 'logical' constructs for the terrifying emotions, and helps them to understand these emotions and be less at the mercy of their ebb and flow.

There are four functions: attraction (fire), digestion (air), retention (earth) and expulsion (water). Attraction is seen as bringing into the body all that it needs in terms of food, water, air, etc; digestion is the separating and assimilating of these substances; retention is the storage and refining;

and expulsion is the act of getting rid of waste from the body.

There are also four realms: imagination (fire), feeling (water), thought (earth) and judgement (air). Imagination is the ability to intuit the future; feeling to relate emotionally; thinking to analyse rationally and judgement to see issues from a wider perspective.

Throughout the book I have used the traditional system of medical astrology which predates the discovery of the so called trans-Saturnian planets: Uranus (discovered in 1781), Neptune (1846) and Pluto (1930). For this reason, none of the plants mentioned are ruled by these planets, neither are these planets included in the humoural system. Modern astrologers have tried to 'place' these planets in the physical body. I am for the most part unhappy about this; most of the information seems speculative and repetitious. Thus some of the material in this book may be at variance with contemporary astrological thinking.

Each of the seven planets (that is, the Sun, Moon, Mercury, Venus, Mars, Saturn and Jupiter) have specific and individual characteristics. They also have qualities in common. The Sun and Mars are hot and dry, and have the qualities of fire: action, intuition, burning, energy. They are associated with the choleric humour, and signify illness such as fevers, itchy rashes, burning, stabbing pains, any condition where the body feels hot and dry. The Sun rules the heart and the vital spirit of the body, that is, the energy which each person is born with, the circulation of the blood, together with the eyesight. Mars rules the gall bladder, red blood cells, the sense of smell and the muscles. Venus and the Moon are cold and moist. They have the qualities of water: receptivity, feeling, cooling and blending. They are associated with the phlegmatic humour, and show illnesses such as catarrh, discharges, accumulations of fluid in the body, menstrual problems and any illness where the body is cold and damp. The Moon rules the fluids in the body, such as the lymph glands, tears, and breast milk, as well as the menstrual cycle and womb. Venus rules the reproductive organs in the woman, the complexion and the hair, the kidneys and the veins. Mercury and Saturn have the qualities of coldness and dryness and are associated with the element earth. Earth provides structures, is slow moving, sensation-orientated and cooling. Saturn rules the bones, the ears, the teeth, the spleen and the skin. Mercury rules the brain and nervous system, reflexes, sight, the thyroid gland and respiration. The melancholic humour rules depression and illnesses associated with the brain, the bones, hearing, the nervous system and breathing. Jupiter represents the element air and its qualities of expansion, lightness, thinking, warmth and moisture. The humour is sanguine and is concerned with conditions of growth (benign and otherwise), digestion, dispersion and nutrition. Jupiter rules the liver, fat cells, blood plasma, the hip joints and growth. Examples of sanguine illnesses include obesity, anorexia, liver disease, benign and cancerous growths.

Each of the herbs is ruled by a planet and has its characteristics or virtues. A herb treats illnesses ruled by the planet. Herbs ruled by Venus, for example, are often used to treat menstrual problems, and herbs of Mercury treat the lungs. In discovering the affiliation of each herb to its planet a deeper understanding of the nature of the plant is possible.

For the purpose of this book, a person's Sun sign or Moon sign (if known) will provide clues to the most suitable remedy.[3]

The word *chakra* comes from the Sanskrit, meaning wheel. Chakras are energy centres found in the etheric body. The etheric body is the term used to describe the energy field which surrounds the physical body and is its template. For example, physical illnesses can be seen in the etheric body, or aura, before they appear in the physical body. The seven chakras are connecting points in the etheric body where different kinds of energies collect and are expressed. Herbs work on individual chakras, some working on several.

The first three chakras reside below the diaphragm. The

base chakra, at the base of the spine, is concerned with survival instincts, security and grounding. Many roots work from this chakra, pulling the energy downwards, stabilising and centring. Examples include comfrey, liquorice, juniper and bearberry. The next chakra, for women, is the womb. Here the energies of reproduction and sexuality are expressed. The Chinese say a woman's soul is here. Physically and emotionally, issues concerned with childbearing, fertility and creativity are expressed in the womb. Pennyroyal and lady's mantle act on this chakra. The solar plexus chakra is concerned with communication and expression of 'gut' feelings: fear, anger, passion and desire. (The solar plexus, a network of nerve tissues and fibres, resides at the pit of the stomach.) Many of our everyday relationships operate from here. Herbs of the solar plexus include chamomile, dandelion, lavender and centaury.

These first three chakras are said to be concerned with our more instinctual nature, our survival mechanisms, the more 'selfish' range of human emotions. Chakras are said to be opened or closed. For most people, the three below the diaphragm are open.

The four chakras above the diaphragm, the heart, throat, third eye and crown chakras, express energies of a more collective, integrated type. The heart chakra is about love, impersonal love. We express this chakra when we feel and express the more profound human emotions: joy, compassion, acceptance. Remedies which work with the heart chakra include rosemary, melissa, hawthorn and lime flowers. The throat chakra is concerned with self-expression and creativity. There is a connection with this chakra and the womb. Sexuality can be expressed as a purely reproductive impulse or as the greatest and most intimate of human experiences. Working magically with sexuality involves the raising of energies from the womb to the throat chakra. Plants include sage and centaury. The chakra in the middle of the forehead, the brow chakra, the third eye, is concerned with vision, clear seeing, clairvoyance and will. People who meditate are opening and developing this chakra. Witchcraft and other magical work can be performed from here. Mugwort is the best known herb for this. The seventh chakra, the crown chakra, or thousand petalled lotus, relates to our divinity. This is where spiritual energies enter the aura. Situated at the top of the head, this is the last chakra to open. Spiritual beings, the Buddha, Christ, saints and mystics, are often depicted with a glowing light here. Meadowsweet enhances the activity of the crown chakra. Our spiritual evolution can be seen as a journey through these seven focal points.

This is a European herbal, in part because I am a European, albeit with strong links to the continents of Africa and Asia, but also because I felt it was important to put the European philosophical beliefs alongside the more developed systems of the Americas, India, Asia and Africa. Not with the aim to show that one perspective is of more value or interest than another, but for the sake of completeness. I believe that if the different systems are studied, common themes will emerge, that is, theories of health and disease which carry around the world. These may change because of cultural and climactic conditions, but I expect a general agreement will be found on the cause of illnesses. Astrology, for example, is found in the healing traditions of India, China and the Americas. The astrology may differ but the principles remain constant and a connection is made with the movements of the planetary bodies and health. The elements, whether three, four or five, are also a common source of reference. What struck me, as a new practitioner of herbal medicine, was the absence of a European tradition. Had there been one? If so, where had it gone? And why had it disappeared? The answers to these questions led me to study herbal and astrological history.

Clearly there had once been a herbal tradition, the last important writings on which occurred around the middle of the sixteenth century in Europe, notably in the work of Nicholas Culpeper. Had there been a woman's tradition? Reading *A History of Women in Medicine* by K C Hurd-Mead and M Lipinska's *Histoire des femmes medicinal*, as well as Lindsay River and Sally Gillespie's *Knot of Time*, it was clear there had in fact been women physicians for millennia. (I write about this is my own *History of Women Healers*, to be published by The Women's Press in 1992.) From the queens of Egypt 6000 BP[4] to Greek and Roman women, including Trotula, a herbalist who practised and lectured at the great medical school at Salerno, to Hildegard of Bingen[5] and the women physicians in mediaeval France excommunicated for practising medicine.[6] At one time in Europe the idea of a woman doctor was neither strange nor unusual, and although many of them have not left written records of their work[7] it is clear from contemporary writings that they did exist and that their practices flourished. So what happened?

There was the witchcraze. Between the fourteenth and sixteenth centuries AD, there was a public campaign against witches in Europe, spearheaded by the Catholic Church but also supported and encouraged by the legal and medical professions. In 1484 The *Malleus Maleficarum* was published.[8] Europe was in turmoil. Not only had an estimated one-third of the population died from the plague but the old social order was crumbling. New alliances were being made and the rich and ambitious were bidding for power. The richest and most influential force at the time was the Church, which itself was in disarray. There was an internal struggle taking place between those who believed in poverty and unworldliness and those who were interested in secular power. There were also popular revolts against the strict rules of the church, and 'witch' was to those times what 'Communist' was to the West until recently. A campaign was organised, fuelled by both religious zeal and the need to find scapegoats, a campaign of such ferocity that Matilda Gage[9] estimates nine million witches were put to death in Europe in the three centuries that followed. The vast majority of these 'witches' were women. Some were probably innocent older women, single women, 'difficult' women[10] and many of these were healers, herbalists and midwives.

A very complex system was developed to determine whether or not a woman was a witch, had been bewitched or was using witchcraft. In all cases the final word lay with the Church, the law and the medical profession. Illnesses which could not be treated by male physicians were said to have been caused by witchcraft, and if such an illness should be cured by anyone other than a male physician, the cure had to be through diabolic means, that is, with the aid of the forces of evil as perceived by the Church.[11] Midwifery became the focus of great male hysteria and it was said that: 'no one does the Catholic church more harm than the midwife.'[12]

If these women were in any way involved with healing, they would have taken into account the current philosophies and teachings of medicine, in so far as they would have been available to a largely illiterate population. Empirical knowledge would have been passed down from mother to daughter, and no doubt they would have used the phases of the moon and the seasons, if not the more complex sciences of astrology. The humoural system, in everyday use at this time, as can be seen from contemporary literature, would also have been incorporated in their work. Women's knowledge was not often written down and so was not available to outsiders (that is, men). This created a great deal of resentment and jealousy. Such women would have been the modern intuitives: healers, masseurs, herbalists. They would have worked with nature, gently encouraging the vital spirit rather than attacking disease with powerful and deadly remedies. They would have used medicine to mitigate the suffering peculiar to women; they employed painkillers and anaesthetics to help to ease the pain and labour of menstruation and childbirth. This, however, was in direct opposition to the teachings of the Church which maintained that pain and suffering in childbirth was the curse of Eve.

The tradition of women as healers had been in existence

from very early times. Women had been physicians to aristocrats and to fighting troops and had also been wisewomen, midwives and nurses. But from the fourteenth century onwards their rights to study at universities and to study and practice medicine were eroded. At the same time they were under the threat of death if they did anything which could be described as witchcraft. Astrology came under the heading of witchcraft, and in some circles still does today.[13] No wonder, then, that the traditions of herbal medicine 'died', along with its practitioners.[14]

Does this history have any relevance to women healers today? I believe it is of the utmost importance. Women are allowed into the ranks of medicine as long as they are prepared to toe the line. Few 'out' lesbians or radical feminists survive long in any branch of medicine, whether orthodox or complementary, let alone those who choose to work from a more spiritual perspective. If women are allowed into medicine at all, it is only because we are seen to conform to the white, male, Christian orthodoxy.[15]

As healers we know this. As long as we work within patriarchal structures (whether orthodox or complementary) and accept conditions as they are, we are tolerated.[16] But if we push too far, make demands for real change, we see the barriers go down. We become marginalised, silenced by ridicule or contempt; we are starved of cash and resources; we are threatened. Women know this. If we are physicians and healers we have to juggle our consciences within the reality of the market place. We have to learn to negotiate the medical minefield. We have to learn how to keep our integrity as feminists, as lesbians, and how to do the best for both our clients and ourselves. How to nurture and be nurtured; how to break down the artificial barriers which exist between healer and patient; and how to maintain those barriers which are necessary for our own self-protection; and how to balance material gain with intellectual and emotional output. In short, we have to create our politics.

With the burning times as our heritage, we are aware of

the need for caution and circumspection, for we understand that misogyny and homophobia are still very much in evidence. We have to be silent, hidden, careful and yet at the same time be outspoken, fearless and inspired. There is much unravelling to be done in our common European history and many wounds to heal. The process will be long and painful. Our work as healers can be seen as a revolutionary act.

Contact with nature, that is, how we notice, feel for and work with our natural surroundings, is our life blood. As women we are connected to the ebb and flow of the seasons by the tidal nature of our own rythms. Our ability to move and adapt from one situation to the next is inherent. Our menstrual cycles demand that in the course of one short lunar month we change, shift and melt into different realities and embrace different experiences. We have a closer, more emphathetic tie to nature and her rhythms than men.

Herbs are the legacy which was left to us by our wise foremothers. Even within the most polluted city, plants flourish, growing by the sides of roads, peeking out from brickwork or tarmac. Their tenacity is awesome and their adaptability a lesson to all of us who feel alienated and frightened by the way we live now. Plants give life to the dead highways and byways of our land, they open our hearts and make our spirits soar. In times of grief the sight of a bud bursting into life can give hope of happier times. They are our wise companions on this planet and they have much to teach us.

Notes

1. Dr Edward Bach realised that many of the physical ailments he was treating had their basis in the emotions. The remedies are discussed at length in Philip Chancellor, *Handbook of the Bach Flower Remedies*, Daniel, London, 1971.

2. Culpeper was a herbalist and an astrologer who practised in and around London in the 1650s. He was a man of the people and championed the cause of the lay healer. The College of Physicians, the ruling body of medicine, tried to discredit him but failed to do so.

3. For an explanation of which planets rule what signs, refer to *The Knot of Time*, by Lindsay River and Sally Gillespie.

4. BP= Before the Present. This is a method of dating which does not use Christianity as a main source of reference.

5. Hildegard of Bingen (1098-1179), known as the Sibyl of the Rhine, was Abbess of Rupertsberg Abbey, near Bingen. She wrote fourteen books, including *De Simplicic Medicinae* and *Causae et Curae*.

6. For example, Jacoba Felice, born in 1280, who was charged with illegally practising medicine, was found guilty and prohibited from working under pain of excommunication. There was no evidence of medical malpractice produced at her trial in 1322; her crime was simply to have been a woman physician.

7. There are few medical books written by women, partly because many women were unable to write, education being denied them, and partly because books that were known to have been written by women have been lost or destroyed. Most of the works of Trotula, for example, which are mentioned in contemporary writings, have not survived.

8. The *Malleus Maleficarum* was a document published by two monks outlining the way a witch could be identified, and heralded the beginning of a campaign of terror against witches – who in fact might simply have been anyone opposed to the Catholic church.

9. See Matilda Gage, *Women, Church and State*, first published in 1893, second edition published by Arno Press, New York, 1972.

10. *Smeddum* was a Scottish term used to describe witches and women who were wild and difficult to control. See C. Larner, *The Witch Hunt in Scotland*.

11. See the *Malleus Maleficarum*, part I, Q II.

12. See The Rev. Montague Summer, *Malleus Maleficarum*, Pushkin Press, 1928, pp. 45-6.

13. 'I read with incredulity the attempt by some . . . to reverse the

clock and drag our profession back into the dark ages of superstition, astrology and alchemy. The successful struggle to free medical herbalism from this incubus of darkness . . .' This quotation is taken from *Greenleaves*, the journal for the National Institute of Medical Herbalists, in December 1988. The article was written by F F Hyde, President Emeritus of that body.

14. Cultures do not in fact die. They simply go underground until the time is safe for them to surface again, even though patriarchy would have us believe otherwise.

15. The case of Wendy Savage versus Hackney Health Authority and the disciplinary actions on radical midwives is very relevant in this respect. See, for instance, *Nursing Times*, 8 June 1988, vol 84, no 23, pp 16-18: '. . . of the 20 registered independent midwives (most of whom work in London), 7 have been subject to disciplinary action in the last year.'

16. Here it is worth noting that the same patriarchal structures exist within complementary (that is, alternative) medicine as they do within mainstream medicine. Unfortunately they are only alternative in the sense that they are different disciplines. Many think complementary medicine is anti-sexist and anti-racist. This is far from the truth.

PART 2

THE HERBAL

The herbal is arranged so that each herb is classified under one of the seven planets. I felt this was the best way of organising the information to show the strong relationship between astrology and herbal medicine.

It will be seen that all herbs ruled by a particular planet have qualities in common, but that at the same time they have many different ways of working, depending on their individual temperament.

The herbs are described using a more 'three dimensional' approach than that usually found in herbals. That is, that not only are the physical uses described in detail, but the emotional and magical-ritual attributes of herbs are also outlined. Their action on the emotions will come as no surprise to those readers who are familiar with the work of Dr Bach, and I have included correspondences with the energy centres or chakras, and with psychic and spiritual applications where appropriate.

Plants work on all levels. Even if an individual is unaware of their action on the emotional or subtle bodies, changes will occur. People are transformed by plants in ways both obvious and subtle.

In my esoteric plant workshops over the past ten years, I have found that plants are a repository for memories. The women participants almost always picked up similar, if not identical, information, changed only in emphasis peculiar to the individual woman. Working with plants in this way enables women to understand their deeper nature and to go far beyond dry academic explanations of their virtues.

Information of many kinds can be collected, and because the plants are as individual as the women participants, some plants will have affinity with some women and will reveal their deepest mysteries, while others which feel out of tune with the woman concerned will reveal very little.

Plants contain the wisdom of their culture. They are teachers. By tuning into them psychically, knowledge can be gleaned about the plants themselves and about the culture to which they belong.

Visualisation for psychically working with plants
I have used this visualisation in my magical herbalism workshops, and much of the psychic and emotional uses of plants emerged from this work. The intention is to penetrate deep into the 'aura' of the plant to find information, and connect in with the wisdom of the plant in ways other than intellectually.

Find a quiet spot where you will be undisturbed for about thirty minutes.

Sit comfortably and take a few deep breaths. Allow your body to relax, slowly letting go of everyday thoughts and preoccupations. Allow yourself to contact that quiet, clam inner space.

Gently open your eyes and pick up the plant to be worked with. (Use a freshly picked sample, if at all possible, although dried herbs can be used even though they do not work so well.)

Hold the plant and look carefully at it, as though seeing it for the first time. Look at its structure, its shape, how the leaves and flowers are arranged. Notice any scent, any colours. Without thinking, allow sensations and feelings to arise which talk about the plant to you. Then taste a bit of the plant. Feel its flavour, how its taste reacts in your mouth and whether there are any physical sensations associated with its taste. Move really slowly through this process, allowing your physical senses to intuit, to gather knowledge.

Then close your eyes, still holding the plant, and allow

your consciousness to move deeper into the plant. If this plant were a person, imagine what she would be like, and allow an image to build for this plant 'fairy'. Take your time. Eventually she will emerge. Allow her to lead you through her mysteries. Here you may see a number of images, feel physical and emotional sensations, hear sounds. Simply remember what comes up and move on to the next thing. Often the images seem to make no sense until they are connected with the whole experience, so at this stage, don't try to understand – just experience. The fairy might lead you to a particular place; follow her if it feels right.

Be aware that with any psychic/magical work, should you feel afraid or want to stop, you can do so whenever you want to. You are always in charge of your experience.

When you feel ready, come back into the room, back into your body and the 'ordinary' world, and write down your experiences. Afterwards you can look up the uses of the plant and check out your work.

I have found this work is best done in groups, so that women can exchange and compare notes.

The exercise can be repeated to gain ever deeper insight into the plant. Try it with a number of plants to widen your field of knowledge.

For reasons of space, the esoteric, that is, the magical and ritual and emotional sections, are limited to what I considered to be the most salient and relevant points.

Like other forces in nature, plants need to be respected for their mystery and power and approached in the correct spirit.

In any method of divination, the mind-set of the enquirer is the pivotal force which will determine sucess or failure in the undertaking.

I hope this book provides a taste of the potential use of plants and where, if we leave our prejudices and fear of the unknown behind, they are able to lead us.

A herb can be any plant material: root, berry, leaves, stem, flowers or bark – anything which is used for medicinal purposes. Nettle is a herb, so is parsley, hawthorn berries and slipepry elm bark. A more scientific name for a herb is medicinal plant. The possible confusion with the term 'herb' arises because herbs are usually seen to flavour food.

The herbs in this book are not dangerous to use unless otherwise specified. The reader is the best judge of her own health and she is encouraged to act responsibly when trying out the remedies. Herbs have their limitations, as do all other forms of medicine, but in my experience there are few side effects found in allopathic medicine compared to those found when using conventional chemical medicine.

Medicine is very political and drug companies wield a great deal of power, as do the professional bodies controlling the practices of doctors and pharmacists. This must be borne in mind when yet another herb poisoning scare occurs. It would appear that much of the hysteria engendered around the toxic effects of plants is more related to those who prescribe these than the herbs themselves.

Remember that for women to self-medicate is for women to take power for themselves. I see the use of plant medicine as a seditious act; plants grow everywhere – we can all use them and lessen our dependence on the orthodox system of chemical medical practice.

1
HERBS OF THE SUN

Element: *Fire*

Organ: *Heart*

Realm: *Imagination*

Humour: *Choleric*

Function: *Attraction*

Qualities: *Hot and dry*

Solar herbs support the vital spirit, the essential energy of the body, which may be compared with the Qi of the Chinese or Prana in the Indian traditions. As Culpeper states, 'regard the heart, keep that upon the wheels, because the Sun is the foundation of life'.[1]

The herbs of the Sun included in this book are: centaury, chamomile, juniper, marigold and rosemary.

CENTAURY

Planetary ruler: *Sun*

Qualities: *Hot and dry*

Harvest time: *July*

Parts used: *Aerial*

Scientific name: *Erythraea centarium*

Medicinal uses: *For the liver and the blood*

Main constituents: *Bitters, valeric acid,
resin, essential oil*

Myths and legends
The name 'Centaury' is said to relate to Chiron the centaur, who was reputed to have healed a wound poisoned by the blood of a hydra. The ancients called it *fel terrae*, gall of the earth, which related to its bitterness. In southern counties of England the herb was known as the centre of the Sun.

Saxon herbalists prescribed it for snake bites and for the treatment of intermittent fever, hence the name feverwort.

Physical uses
Centaury purges choler from the body and increases the flow of bile from the liver and gall bladder as a result of its bitterness. It can therefore be used for all illnesses which affect those organs: gall stones, jaundice, hepatitis, nausea, lack of appetite, sluggish digestion, indigestion and any kind of parasites. It helps in intermittent fevers, post-viral syndrome and viruses. It rids the body of accumulated water due to liver disease (hepatic oedema).

Use in cases of gout, rheumatism and muscle cramps as a blood cleanser. Centaury brings on delayed periods and helps womb pains in general, including after-birth pain and cramps. It has a general sedative action on the nervous system. As a potent blood purifyer, Centaury is most helpful in skin erruptions, eczema and boils. As a solar herb it is helpful to the eyes, for both inflammation and weakness of sight. Centaury strengthens the heart and keeps the vital spirit up.

Centaury is used as a Bach flower remedy and is prescribed for people who are timid and fearful and who need to please others. They easily become dominated by more forceful characters as they themselves are submissive. They tend towards martyrdom and masochistic relationships.

Recipe
Trotula's recipe for retention of the period

    5 g (⅛ oz) myrrh
    5 g (⅛ oz) centaury
    5 g (⅛ oz) sage

Powder finely and add 2½ g (¹⁄₁₆ oz - 1 dram) of the mixture to a tisane of nettle and myrrh.

    Dose: Drink freely.

Emotional uses
Centaury works on the solar plexus and throat chakras. The herb is related to the expression of rage, self justified rage, the 'I am worth more than this' kind of emotion. It is about not letting other people stomp all over you, and standing up for your rights. Not quite the warrior aspect, more the tigress, who defends her own with primal ferocity.

Take a tisane of centaury first thing in the morning, so that you can face the day with courage.

Centaury is useful for watery types who too easily offer themselves up for sacrifice, often when this is not appropriate. There are many things that are worth standing up for, but this takes courage. The courage to be unpopular, to make a stand against injustice, bigotry and ignorance. A person who takes such action is often alone; the voice of dissention is not a popular one, even if it is saying what many know to be true. We are conditioned by our gender and our culture not to make a fuss, so such a stand is harder still. But this is the way hearts and minds are changed, it is the everyday acts of heroism which influence people's minds.

Magical and ritual uses

Centaury is a herb of the element fire; it represents initiation and intuition. It is drunk before a long journey or where trials of strength are being attempted. Rituals of initiation in wild countryside, among wastelands and mountains where the neophyte must conquer her fear and learn to be at one with the elements. Don Juan of the Castaneda books[2] describes such initiatory rites and his terrain is a familiar one to centaury: magical, inhospitable, ancient, elusive. The Welsh mountains and the Scottish Highlands have such a history and magic, and were the sites of many initiatory ceremonies of Celtic Britain.

Centaury is a herb of the midsummer fires, when women gathered to tell tales of bravery and courage, of ancient battles fought and won.

CHAMOMILE

Planetary ruler: *Sun*

Qualities: *Hot and dry*

Harvest time: *July and August*

Parts used: *Flowers*

Scientific name: *Anthemis nobilis*

Medicinal uses: *For the digestion and nervous disorders*

Main constituents: *Volatile oil, bitters valerianic acid, flavonoids, tannins*

Myths and legends

In the language of flowers, chamomile means patience in adversity. It was known as the herb of humility because, as a lawn plant, the more it was trodden on, the faster it grew.

Chamomile was one of the nine sacred herbs of the Saxons who called it maythen. The plant has a long association with young girls, or nymphs as they are called in the Dianic tradition (that is, witchcraft centred around the goddess Diana).

Maidens were seen to have a special kind of magical power. Their psychic, telepathic and clairvoyant skills were renowned. Often they were used by the older priestesses for scrying with crystal balls and in water (that is, looking into Crystal balls or bodies of water to see images of future events). In initiation rites for young women, they were tested for their obedience and for the fearlessness with which they carried out their tasks. Little is known of the Celtic initiation rites for young women, but it is believed they involved spending time alone (at night) in a sacred grove to contact the spirits there who would help them to find certain magical objects hidden by the initiates. They then had to intuit the religious and magical significance of these objects. Beltane (30 April) was traditionally the time for the initiation of young women. They fasted before the ceremony and during the rite were clad in white robes with golden ornaments. During the festivities which followed, honey cakes were served, honey being sacred to the Goddess. Garlands of spring flowers adorned their hair. Before the rite the girls were bathed in spring water with chamomile flowers in it.

Physical uses

Chamomile is a good, all-round, gentle remedy for both the nervous and digestive systems. Use in any disease of the digestion which is thought to have been caused by nervous tension or anxiety: stomach and duodenal ulcers, heartburn, flatulence, diarrhoea and constipation and irritable bowel syndrome. As it contains a bitter substance, it increases the secretion of digestive juices and the absorption of food. It is a gentle but effective remedy and can be used safely with babies, children and the elderly.

As it relaxes the nervous system, use chamomile for headaches, anxiety, insomnia, palpitations and general fearfulness. In France it is given to children who suffer from nightmares, to make them less fearful. It is also an excellent remedy for teething in babies; use the tea in their bottles or rub a little on the baby's gums to stop the pain. Chamomile is a painkiller and can be used for toothache, earache, neuralgia, and inflamed sores and swellings. As it is the same temperature as blood, that is, the effect on the body is neutral in that it neither heats nor cools, chamomile helps to reduce heat and inflammation, bringing the body temperature back to normal. As a volatile oil it is strongly antiseptic and so can be used wherever there is a need for infections to be countered; it is said to be 120 times stronger than sea water in this respect.

Chamomile has a beneficial action on the womb and can be used for menstrual cramps, for premenstrual tension and to ease the pain of childbirth.

Chamomile is of some help in dealing with allergies, especially asthma and hayfever. As it is a fire herb, it can help to dry up secretions in hayfever and relax the airways in asthma during an attack. It helps to stop sniffles from pollution.

The herb is an excellent remedy for the skin and is widely used to clear up blemishes and to tone the tissues.

For a relaxing bath Tie a handful of chamomile flowers in a muslin bag and fix this underneath the hot water tap. Run the bath in this way and lie in hot water, breathing the steam. Alternatively, if you can afford it, buy essential oil of chamomile and put ten drops of the oil in the hot bathwater. Do not use soap in the water as this will nullify the effect of the oil. For babies and children use two to five drops.
For steam inhalation. Pour boiling water in a large pottery bowl and put five drops of the essential oil or a strong tisane in the water. Cover your head with a towel and breathe in the steam for as long as it is bearable. For an asthma attack and hayfever.

WARNING. Chamomile can be used for mild cases of asthma, but should never be used as a substitute for anti-asthmatic drugs or medical treatment where the condition is serious.

Emotional uses
Chamomile works on the solar plexus chakra. It is very good for either children or adults who have temper tantrums, who express anger which is related to fear and also express the need to protect themselves. It is for people who are prickly, over-sensitive and volatile. Chamomile quietens, relaxes and centres the person, and gives a general sense of well-being, nourishment and security. It is for people who feel emotionally deprived, who feel unloved and uncared for. Chamomile generally helps to ease obstructions, to melt frozen panic or warm up inertia and allows for movement of some kind.

The solar plexus chakra is the place where we take in energy from others. Sometimes we can feel our energy is being sucked out, or that we are under attack from another person. This is almost always an unconscious action on the part of the person attacking; he or she might be very draining or needy and suck the energy of those the individual comes in contact with. There are many who do not have a sense of self, or a strong self-preserving instinct, and they can allow their energy to be leaked in this way and find themselves suffering from headaches, depression, fatigue and listlessness which do not seem to relate to what is happening in their lives. Taken as a tea, used as an oil, or burnt as an incense, whenever you feel in need of nourishment and mothering, chamomile can help to seal off the solar plexus and protect a person from draining people or places. In acute cases, put a few drops of the oil on a yellow silk scarf and tie around the solar plexus.

Magical and ritual uses
Chamomile is an ingredient used in many love potions. It is said that if you wash your hair and face in chamomile you will attract your beloved; another name for chamomile is love apples. To increase passion, sprinkle a little of the tea or flower water on sheets.

Babies traditionally had a small bunch of chamomile hung over their cribs to protect them and keep them free of illness.

Burn chamomile in the room of a dying person to ease their passage into the next world and to counter any fear they might have of letting go.

Chamomile is a good herb to use for girls and young women and can be used in any ritual work to empower them.

JUNIPER

Planetary ruler: *Sun*

Qualities: *Hot and dry*

Harvest time: *Autumn and winter*

Parts used: *Berries*

Scientific name: *Juniperus communis*

Medicinal uses: *For the kidneys and the blood*

Main constituents: *Bitters, tannin, volatile oil, flaronoids, resins*

Physical uses

Jupiter is an excellent remedy to counter any poison taken into the body, or for any toxic or infectious illness. It is a strong acting diuretic, removing excess fluid from the body and increasing the flow of urine. It is a powerful disinfectant and can be used for infections of the urinary tract. It can also be used in kidney stones and gravel to cleanse the system of these particles. Juniper is a deep-acting remedy, which boosts the energy of the vital force and helps to increase vitality after a long illness or depression. Being solar, it counteracts both the fearfulness of phlegmatics and the depression of melancholics. It is an excellent remedy for wind and colic in the body, especially if the berries are eaten in the morning on an empty stomach (ten to twelve berries at a time).

Juniper stimulates the mental processes and is believed to strengthen the sight by fortifying the optic nerves.

As it is a powerful blood cleanser, Juniper is used for arthritis and rheumatism, especially where the disease is caused by cold weather.

The berries may also help to clear up chronic skin disease, especially psoriasis and chronic eczema.

WARNING. Juniper is very powerful and should not be used by people who are very weak and debilitated. Energy should be built up before this remedy is taken. *DO NOT GIVE juniper to pregnant women, children or the frail and elderly.* Take only for three weeks at a time, then rest for three weeks and then take for another three weeks before stopping the treatment. Do not use if the person concerned has serious kidney disease or high blood pressure.

Recipes

2 cups of juniper berries
2 cups of cold pressed oil (eg olive oil)

Soak the berries overnight in water and then simmer for thirty minutes in the oil. Strain.
Apply to itching wounds, the back for back problems, aching joints and sores.

WARNING. Do not drink this mixture.

For Wind and Heartburn
Eat and chew as follows:
4 berries on day 1
5 berries on day 2
6 berries on day 3
7 berries on day 4
and so on, until you are taking 10 berries daily. Then work the numbers back down again to 5.

Kidney Tonic
450g (1lb) fresh dandelion tops and roots
450g (1lb) fresh green peach leaves
450g (1lb) parsley roots and tops
450g (1lb) strawberry vines

Bruise and add 3 gallons (11 litres) of water. Boil and then add: 100 g (4oz) pulverised juniper berries
450g (1lb) sugar.

Allow the mixture to ferment and then strain and bottle for use.

Dose: half a wineglass 4 times daily.

For a prolapsed womb (after Trotula) Make a bath of the following herbs: 10 g (¼ oz) each of mugwort, fleabane, juniper, camphor and wormwood. Sit in this up to the nipples. Use daily. When the womb has retracted, mix 10 g (¼ oz) each of powdered pennyroyal, galangal, spikenhard and muscat grapes together with peppermint oil. Tie into a ball with muslin and use as a plug. Hold in place with a bandage and lie still for several days.

WARNING. Use only under the supervision of a herbal practitioner. Do not self-medicate.

Emotional uses

Juniper is associated with the base chakra, where the Kundalini, or serpent power, lies dormant. It is said that when a certain degree of development is achieved, the serpent rises from its slumbering position and pushes upwards through the other chakras, breaking their protective webs and changing the whole energy of the etheric body. Juniper is used for those who are blocked on the physical plane, generally earth types, that is, those with a lot of Taurus, Virgo or Capricorn in their charts. It is also used for those who are looking for a more spiritual way of life, who want to embrace fire. The base chakra is associated with those who are trapped into living only to survive; who cannot, because of fear or hatred or anger, move toward more refined emotional expression. Juniper allows a person to be more detached emotionally and to move on from obsessions or resentments, from anger and violence. Being fiery, juniper can also help to 'dry out' water types, who become lost in a sea of emotion and are unable to act or initiate. Fire provides focus and direction. It energises the will and gives the courage that watery types sometimes lack.

Burn five juniper berries on charcoal at the new and full

moons for three months. Make a note of changes that happen in your spiritual life.

Magical and ritual uses

Kyphi (incense)

To raisins steeped in wine and left for three nights and days, add juniper berries, acacia, henna and calamus root.

Mix the above together and leave for twenty-four hours. Grind in a mortar and add equal parts of this powder to the following mixture, which is also ground in a mortar: mastic, peppermint, bay leaves, hibiscus, cinnamon, gallangal root, orris root and sandlewood.

Mix these well and add powdered myrrh and honey to bind. Spread out on a baking sheet to dry. Burn over a charcoal disc.

To bring more spiritual energies into your life

Starting from the new moon, take time every evening, when the evening star has risen, to burn this incense. As it is burning, meditate on the fire of life which caused the universe to come into existence and keeps our world moving and unfolding. Imagine that spark of light firing the energy which you keep protected in your base chakra. As you meditate,, allow an image to form which represents your spirituality. This image or symbol will give you insights into how your spirituality can be incorporated into your daily life. Allow yourself to become inspired and encouraged by your own spiritual fire.

MARIGOLD

Planetary ruler: *Sun*

Qualities: *Hot and dry*

Harvest time: *August*

Scientific name: *Calendula officinalis*

Medicinal uses: *For the liver, the blood, and gynaecological and bacterial conditions*

Main constituents: *Bitter principle, saponins, sterols, mucilage, gum*

Myths and legends

Marigold was given the Latin name Calendula, after *calends*, the first day of the summer months in the Roman calendar. It was believed to flower on that day.

Marigold was known to be magical. Spanish sorcerers were said to wear it as a talisman. Traditionally it was picked when the Sun entered the sign of Virgo and the picker had to carry a wolf's tooth wrapped in a bayleaf.

In Mexico it is thought to be a flower of death and is believed to have sprung from the blood of the Indians killed by the Spanish invaders.

Henry VIII was reputed to have used marigold mixed with sorrel, burnet, feverfew and snapdragon to combat the plague.

It was said that if you wore marigold flowers you would be able to see who had robbed you.

Xochiquetzal was said to have brought the knowledge of spinning and weaving to the Aztec people, and the gifts of painting and carving and the music of the pipes and drums.

She was the Aztec love goddess of marriage and whores, spinning and weaving, dance and change, magic and art. Her symbols were the dove and the marigold. She was said to have honoured the women who lived for themselves (women-centred women), for Xochiquetzal taught them the power and beauty of their own sensuality and she was said to delight in women's sexual pleasure. Xochiquetzal taught her people the message of the marigold, the petalled book of the cycles of life, of seed to leafy stem, of leafy stem to bud, of bud to flower open to the Sun, of flower to drying petals that were the womb for the seed – to complete the cycle. In this way the Aztecs were taught the flow of life eternal, and the interconnectedness of all things. Xochiquetzal was seen as Goddess of the land of the dead and her statues were honoured on the day of the dead ones, and the offerings of marigold petals were made to her.

Physical uses

Marigold is a potent liver remedy and as such is the choice remedy in all illnesses affecting the liver, or caused by the liver malfunctioning. Use in jaundice, hepatitis and cirrhosis. Use also as a digestive stimulant, for lack of appetite, poor digestion, which often results in smelly feet, and absorption, constipation, wind and peptic ulcers. It is a powerful healing remedy and helps to heal wounds in the digestive tract such as ulcers, colitis and diverticulitis.

As it is powerful blood cleanser, I have used marigold with great success in cases of chronic eczema, boils, acne and teenage spots. It works on the lymphatic system and so is used for swollen lymph glands, tonsilitis, chronic sore throats and where the immune system of the body has lowered resistance. Use for viral and fungal infections.

Dian Buchman in *Herbal Medicine* (p. 29) describes how Dr Petire Hoyle used marigold almost exclusively for dressing wounds in his front-line hospital in the First World War and how he was commended for the clean state of his patients' wounds. She also writes about Dr Dorothy Shephard who used the tincture during the Blitz in London during the Second World War to dress wounds and found that it prevented infection in a way other antiseptics were unable to.

Marigold has a special affinity for the reproductive

system and is used for regulating irregular periods, to treat chronic thrush and other vaginal infections, and to heal any wounds caused by, for example, abortions, miscarriages and any surgery in the gynecological area such as ovarian cysts, polyps and pelvic inflammatory disease. It is also used as a healing agent after a traumatic delivery or caesarian section. Marigold is one of the remedies I use for any problems with the cervix: inflamed cervix, abnormal smears and erosions. (With abnormal smears, it is best to consult a herbal practitioner. See also, *Our Bodies, Ourselves*, published by the Boston Women's Health Book Collective.)

Deep cuts can be treated by using marigold.

This is a safe herb to take in pregnancy. In the treatment of premenstrual awareness (PMA),[3] Marigold can help relieve the symptoms of irritability, water retention, skin erruptions and thrush by stimulating the action of the liver and speeding up the breakdown of hormones. PMA may be due to abnormal secretion of hormones, but more commonly I have found it is because the liver fails to break down the hormones, so they stay in the bloodstream for longer and at a higher level and cause the symptoms. If it is the liver that is at fault here, using marigold for two menstrual cycles will clear up this problem.

Marigold is the best remedy for varicose veins, and may be used both internally and externally as an astringent. It helps to restore tone to the veins and eases the circulation.

Use Marigold for eye infections. As a solar herb, it is an excellent remedy for conjunctivitis, and used as an eye bath it will clear up the infection without the need for antibiotics.

Recipes
Marigold Ointment
>500 ml (18 fl oz) of infused marigold oil
>(see preparation section p. 222ff.)
>40 g (1½) cocoa butter
>40 g (1½) yellow beeswax

Gently warm the oil, taking care not to boil it. Melt in the cocoa butter and beeswax, remove from the heat and stir until cool and thick. Store in glass jars. If the weather is very hot, store in the fridge.

Use for wounds, infected grazes, athletes foot and burns after the heat has gone out of them.

Marigold Douche
>   80 ml (2¾ fl oz) rosewater
>   10 ml (1 teasp) marigold tincture
>   10 ml (1 teasp) comfrey tincture

Mix all the ingredients and shake well. (The mixture will keep indefinitely.)

Dose: 10 ml (1 teaspoon) in 1 cup of warm water as a douche, for thrush, cystitis, etc.

Eye Bath and Skin Wash
>   50 ml (2 fl oz) rosewater
>   40 ml (1¾ fl oz) witch hazel
>   1 ml (1 teasp) marigold tincture

Mix and soak cotton wool pads in the liquid.

Apply to sore, red eyes, or to pimples and boils – it will draw out the poison from them.

Marigold Conserve: Fill a large earthenware pot with marigold petals and pour on pure honey to cover all the flowerheads completely. Let stand in a warm place for six weeks. Strain. Use for infected wounds – honey is a powerful antiseptic – and give to children with infectious diseases such as chicken pox.

Dose: 10 ml (1 teaspoon) in a cup of warm water three times daily.

Emotional uses

Marigold is said to comfort the heart and spirit. It is used for people who are nervous and easily frightened, who have low defences, pick up illnesses easily and feel themselves in need of protection. It is associated with shock and trauma and the expression of strong emotions, particularly anger. A solar herb, marigold is used to temper the excesses of Mars; that is, anger, impatience and pent up energy. It is good for hot-headedness; in the form of headaches with stabbing pains and for rashness, intolerance and foolhardiness. It has a smoothing effect, like that of unruffling feathers and soothes prickliness.

Buy some marigold flowers and keep them wrapped in a white cloth. Carry them with you. When you feel in need of protection, hold the bag and feel the warm solar energy radiating through you.

Magical and ritual uses

There is too much Mars energy in the world today, which marigold can help to balance out. There is aggression which is expressed in the world and aggression we direct at ourselves. Eating polluted foods, smoking and drinking alcohol are ways in which we take out our frustration on ourselves. The body is the temple we inhabit; it can be cleansed twice yearly with fasts and by drinking the tea of marigold flowers. Eat less and eat well; we should try to cut out pollutants from our lives: cosmetics, harmful chemicals. We need to connect again with the solar life-giving forces; we need to live with nature, co-operating with each other to stop the deadly road we are travelling down. The sun is reborn each day; we can give birth to a new way of living, a new world.

ROSEMARY

Planetary ruler: *Sun*

Qualities: *Hot and dry*

Harvest time: *May to September*

Parts used: *Leaves and flowers*

Scientific name: *Rosmarinus officinalis*

Medicinal uses: *For the heart, the digestion and nervous disorders*

Main constituents: *Volatile oil, tannins, resins, camphor*

Myths and legends

Students studying in ancient Greece used to entwine rosemary twigs in their hair to improve their memories.

At the time of the Black Death, the herb was burnt indoors to prevent the risk of contagion and was used in churches as a cheap substitute for incense. Mourners at funerals carried a sprig of rosemary to prevent infection from the corpse and threw the sprigs into the grave with the coffin to prevent the spread of disease. It was burnt with juniper berries in sick rooms and hospitals to prevent contagion.

Rosemary was an emblem of fertility and was used in marriage festivals. In Spain and Italy it was believed to protect the wearer from magical spells. Rosemary leaves put under the bed were supposed to stop bad dreams. Arab physicians put powdered Rosemary on the umbilical cords of newborn infants as an astringent antiseptic.

Rosemary was a charm against snake bites and the stings of venemous insects. The leaves and flowers were tied in a small bag and hung around the necks of children.

There was a superstition that where Rosemary blossomed

in a garden the woman was the head of the household. Apparently men were believed to secretly damage the bushes lest they be ridiculed for their lack of power.

Physical uses
Rosemary is a stimulant to the nervous system and, being hot and dry, is useful where the body is cold and sluggish and needs pepping up to dispel cold and phlegm, one of the four humours. Use for depression, lethargy, dizzyness, poor memory and concentration and migraine due to feeling cold, and any disease of excess phlegm. Rosemary increases the blood flow to the head and helps concentration and wakefulness. It is useful as a stimulant for complicated mental tasks when caffeine has to be avoided.

WARNING. If there is a history of high blood pressure, it is best not to take rosemary during pregnancy. Consult a herbalist for advice.

As a solar herb it is a heart tonic and strengthens the action of the heart, causing it to beat more strongly, whilst increasing the circulation of blood, so the herb is especially for those with cold limbs, chilblains and poor circulation. It will raise low blood pressure. It is a digestive and liver remedy and is especially useful for wind, colic and indigestion and the bloated feeling after meals. It helps to digest fatty or rich foods.

Rosemary has been used as a remedy and as a preventative against hardening of the arteries or arteriosclerosis.

Recipes
Tea for Arteriosclerosis
Equal parts of: rosemary, lavender, mint and yarrow.
Take one cup twice daily before meals.

Queen of Hungary water
450 g (1lb) of rosemary flowers
3½ litres (1 gallon) of white wine

Soak the flowers in the wine for one month.

Apply to the paralysed part.

The Queen of Hungary was said to have cured herself of paralysis using this lotion on her limbs.

Oil of Rosemary

    120 ml (4 fl oz) sunflower oil
    100 drops of essential oil of rosemary

Massage into the limbs of stroke patients who have suffered paralysis. Use regularly for at least six months. Some sensation may return to the limbs. (This recipe was given to me by an aromatherapist friend who claimed she had seen significant results using this treatment.)

Rosemary Wine

    1 bottle white wine
    1 handful of fresh (or 2 x 15ml (tbsp) of dried)
    rosemary leaves
    2 x 15 ml (tbsp) dried borage leaves

Steep herbs in the wine for two weeks.

Take a small wineglassful when your spirits need lifting or for mild depression.

Emotional uses

Rosemary works on the heart chakra and is generally cleansing to the aura, chasing away dark jealous thoughts. It opens the heart and allows the warmth of the midday sun inside, where there is grief, anger, hatred and bitterness. It lets love and joy into the heart. It is for those who have suffered cruelty and abuse at the hands of others such as abused children, battered women and those who have been betrayed or wounded in love. The herb is for those who have high ideals for themselves and for others and who are often disillusioned where, after a time, the disillusionment may turn into bitterness and a wall is built around their hearts to protect themselves. Such people may be capable of doing great cruelty to others because they feel everyone should suffer as they have done. They may be quite cut off from their feelings and immerse themselves in work as a substitute. They may be found in the caring professions, where they take out their bitterness on others.

Conversely, rosemary is also useful for those who are too open hearted and who cannot discriminate amongst people, so that they may collect lame ducks and people who bask in their light and drain their energy. These may also be seen in the helping professions, but they can easily get burnt out and exhausted. Here there is a need to have a stronger sense of self-worth, to temper the selflessness with some discrimination so that the greatest benefit may be obtained from their work.

Make a bath of rosemary - 1 x 15 ml (table)spoonful of the herb in a cotton bag - or use 5 drops of the essential oil. Lie in this for ten to fifteen minutes.

Magical and ritual uses
For regulating the heart chakra
Burn rosemary as an incense. Focus your attention on a spot between your shoulder blades and allow an image to come of the heart chakra. Hold this image in your mind, allowing golden sunlight to stream into it, warming and strengthening it. Be aware of how you open and close this chakra and practise a few times, feeling how it is to be fully open, half open and closed. Notice any difficulties you experience and any feelings this brings up for you. Do this daily for a month. Keep a diary of how you feel and the effect this meditation has had on your emotional life.

Notes
1. Nicholas Culpeper, *The English Physician, englarged*, p. 395.
2. Don Juan, a Yaqui man of knowledge, trained Carlos Casteneda in the shamanic traditions of the Mexican indians. He is described in detail in Casteneda's many books, for example, *The Teachings of Don Juan* (1979) and *A Separate Reality* (1980).
3. I use the term 'premenstrual awareness' rather than the more

usual 'premenstrual tension' to get away from the notion of sickness and incapacity. The time immediately before a period for a woman is one of change, difference, awareness, of sensing things in other world and time.

2
HERBS OF VENUS

Element: *Water*

Organs: *womb, skin, hair, kidneys, and throat*

Realm: *Feeling*

Humour: *Phlegmatic*

Function: *Expulsion*

Qualities: *Cold and moist*

Of all the herbs, those of Venus are the most plentiful. If you think of all the life-giving properties associated with this planet, it is not surprising her plants should feature so strongly in the herbalist's collection. Generally speaking, herbs of Venus are soothing, calming, gently expulsive and cleansing. Although the individual herbs will be differing degrees of heat and dryness, the overall qualities of Venus are strong in these herbs.

The herbs of Venus included in this book are: coltsfoot, cowslip, elderflower, lady's mantle, mugwort, pennyroyal, thyme and vervain.

COLTSFOOT

Planetary ruler: *Venus*

Qualities: *Warm and moist*

Harvest time: *Flowers
in February; leaves in
March*

Parts used: *Flowers
and leaves*

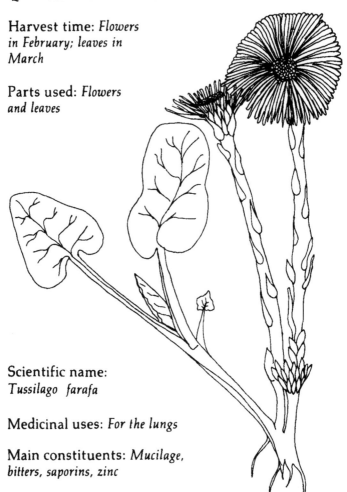

Scientific name:
Tussilago farafa

Medicinal uses: *For the lungs*

Main constituents: *Mucilage,
bitters, saporins, zinc*

Myths and legends

The botanical name, *tussilago*, means cough disperser, from the Latin *tussis*, meaning cough. And *lago* in Latin means 'I carry' (away).

Coltsfoot used to be the apothecaries' painted sign and hung above their shops.

Physical uses

Coltsfoot is one of the main remedies for the lungs, and is usually found in herbal cough mixtures sold over the counter at health food stores. The mucilage has the effect of soothing a dry, irritating cough, and helping phlegm trapped in the lungs to be coughed up. It can be used with quick results for acute bronchitis. It is soothing to the throat and larynx and so can be given when there is tonsilitis and laryngitis. As it contains the mineral zinc, the herb has the effect of healing damaged and diseased tissues and can therefore be used with some degree of success to heal the lesions of tuberculosis and emphysema, and can minimise the amount of scarring which results. I have used coltsfoot with great success in cases of whooping cough; it relaxes the lungs and helps the tough mucus to be expelled. Whooping cough treated herbally, in my experience, resolves far quicker than if treated with conventional medicines. Coltsfoot helps to expel tar, dust, and other pollutants from the lungs and is given to smokers to minimise the effects of tobacco smoke. Anyone who has to work in a polluted environment, cyclists in cities or those who are allergic to dust, would be advised to take a weekly dose of coltsfoot to clear debris from their lungs. Smokers or recent ex-smokers would also benefit from a regular cup of coltsfoot tea to minimise damage from the irritant smoke. Tobacco is a herb of Mars, and therefore a hot and dry herb which has the effect of drying out the moisture from the lungs and making them more susceptible to infection and growths. Coltsfoot counters the irritation.

By making mucus in the lungs more fluid, coltsfoot acts as a decongestant and can be used to treat colds and coughs, particularly where there is a fear that the infection might spread to the lungs. Because of its relaxing qualities, coltsfoot can also be used to help relieve constriction in the lungs associated with asthma and breathlessness. In asthma especially, it relieves spasm of the airways and at the same time makes the mucus more fluid, preventing the formation of plugs of thick mucus which can block the passages.

Externally, coltsfoot flowers can be made into a poultice to treat erysipelas, a red inflamation of the skin, hot rashes and as a wash for varicose ulcers. The leaves and flowers can be made into herbal tobacco which can be smoked to stop an acute asthma attack.

Recipes

    15 g (½ oz) coltsfoot leaves
    15 g (½ oz) horehound leaves
    15 g (½ oz) comfrey leaves
    15 g (½ oz) hyssop
    15 g (½ oz) vervain
    1 liquorice stick

Add to 1.75 litres (3 pints) boiling water; stand for thirty minutes.

Dose: 1 5 ml (teaspoon) four to five times daily for coughs.

    25 g (1 oz) coltsfoot leaves
    25 g (1 oz) fennel
    10 g (¼ oz) fresh ginger root

Add 900 ml (1½ pints) boiling water, simmer and reduce liquid to 300 ml (½ pint) and add 225 g (½ lb) honey.

Dose: 1 x 5 ml (teaspoon) three to four times a day for coughs, chills and catarrh.

To cool a hot fever (after Culpeper)

Mix equal parts of elder and coltsfoot flowers and add a pinch of meadowsweet. Make into a strong decoction, 25 g (1 oz) to 600 ml (1 pint), and simmer for fifteen minutes.

Dose: 1 tablespoon three to five times a day in warm water.

British herbal tobacco

Mix 10 grams (¼ oz) of each of the following according to taste: coltsfoot, buckbean, eyebright, betony, rosemary, thyme, lavender and chamomile.

Smoke for asthma, bronchitis and other lung complaints. Smoking herbs in this way does not have the same bad effects as smoking tobacco.

Emotional uses

As it is related to the solar plexus, coltsfoot is drawn by its inherent quality of lightness and clearness to its opposite, that is, darkness and heaviness. Coltsfoot expels tar and other accumulations in the lungs and it works to remove similar emotional debris. Envy blocks out the light; sunlight can not filter through its darkness as it deadens the life force and drags the spirit down, creating dullness and heaviness. Emotions such as envy and jealousy, which cannot and will not be expressed via the throat, become stuck in the lungs and can, after many years, cause the tissues to become corroded and eaten away. Serious illness then develops. These strong emotions can devour the body from the inside. Coltsfoot is a remedy for thin people with black hair and dark complexions. Those who hold on to bitterness. Conversely, those who deny reality, who will not acknowledge their darker side, their shadow, whose fear of darkness and chaos is enormous, and are constantly on the run from their own inner darkness, must, at all costs, embrace the light. They should also take coltsfoot.

Make a tea of coltsfoot and drink it at the end of each day for a lunar month (that is, from full moon to full moon). Repeat on alternate months if you feel the need.

Magical and ritual uses

Coltsfoot can work to clear channels for vision, for clarity, for far-seeing. Coltsfoot can be used to help clairvoyance, and can be drunk as a tea, or burnt as incense. It has a focusing, purifying quality, allowing for messages and intuitions to come through.

COWSLIP

Planetary ruler:
Venus

Qualities:
Warm and moist

Harvest time:
April and May

Parts used:
Flowers

Scientific name:
Primula veris

Medicinal uses:
*For the lungs
and nervous disorders*

Main constituents:
*Saporins, essential
oils, glycosides*

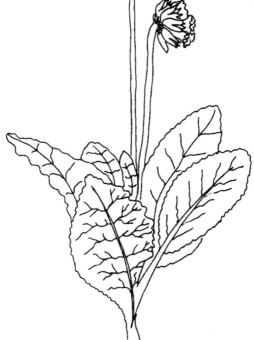

Myths and legends

One of cowslip's old names was key flower which refers to its association to the Norse Goddess, Freya, and the flowers were thought to admit one to her treasure palace. Freya was the *Vanadis* the ruling ancestress of the *Vanir*, or elder gods, who ruled before the patriarchal god Odin arrived. Odin said he learned all his magic and divine powers from Freya. Freya represented sexual love, and her other name, Frigg, became slang for intercourse. She mated with Frey, the god of Yule, who was then sacrificed to make way for his son, born to Freya. Freya was the mistress of cats, the ruler of fate, the stars and heaven. She was the leader of the Valkyries who led dead warriors to Odin's heaven, Valhalla. Before Odin's time, the Valkyries were amazon warriors who ruled the gates of death. The Valkyries were also the Mare-women, and like the ancient horse-masked priestesses of Demeter they could carry a man away to his death. Valkyries were considered identical to witches during the middle ages and one source claims there were thirteen Valkyries, the number of witches needed for a coven.

Cowslip is a favourite of old herbals. Women would come into London and sell them in bunches in street corners, in the same way as violets were sold, and they were believed to give the wearer luck in love. It was a plant often given to daughters by their fathers and by early courting couples as a tentative start to the long courting rituals.

On may mornings, girls would give each other posies of cowslips and this would be a symbol of trust, of their friendship. Garlands were made of the flowers and dairy cattle hung with them to encourage milk production. Their yellow colour was said to make the butter more creamy and the cheese a more golden colour. In Suffolk, milkmaids would collect cowslips on the morning of May eve (Beltane, 30 April) and mix them with newly collected milk and wash their faces in the mixture, believing it would make their faces glow and attract their beloved in the Beltane celebrations that evening.

Cowslips were the plants of the ordinary working people and were not seen in the salons of the wealthy.

Physical uses

Cowslip is a gentle lung remedy, suitable for babies and small children and the elderly. It is excellent and quick-acting, for feverish colds and flu and mild attacks of bronchitis. It helps to clear the body of poisons. Because it is a sedative, it calms a dry, irritating cough and allows children to sleep through the night without coughing. It can be used for mild insomnia and as a general nerve tonic and relaxant. It strengthens the nerves and stimulates the brain and relieves head aches. In case of neuralgia, an inflamation of the nerves causing pain, it is said to have a beneficial action, and for any kind of nerve pain due to heat or wind. Cowslip helps to cool down heat of the body and to reduce wind (that is, gas or flatulence). The flowers are used to clear blemishes on the skin, reduce acne and are said to prevent wrinkles.

The cowslip is a protected plant, so please buy your cowslip flowers from a reputable supplier rather than pick them from fields or hedgerows.

Recipes

Conserve of cowslip flowers (after Culpeper)

Use only the tender and juicy leaves and flowers. Beat them to a pulp in a mortar until they resemble a thick paste, and to every pound of flowers add 1.5 kg (3 lb) of sugar and beat them very well together. Store in earthenware pots. This mixture will keep for a year.

Dose: a teaspoonful every morning and evening. When in storage, stir occasionally to prevent mould setting in and keep in a cool cellar or fridge to preserve longer.

Cowslip Wine

A gallon of petals with 1.75 kg (4 lb) of lump sugar and the rind of three lemons is added to a gallon of cold spring water. A cup of fresh yeast is added and the liquor stirred every day for a week. It is then put in a barrel with the juice of the three lemons and left to 'work'. When the wine is quiet and has stopped fermenting, cork it down for eight to nine months and then bottle. The wine will be a clear yellow colour and is almost a liqueur.

Given in small doses as a medicine it is helpful for lung infections in babies and small children.

Cowslip Syrup
450 g (1 lb) of fresh flowers. Infuse in 900 ml (1½ pints) of boiling water and simmer with loaf sugar to make a yellow syrup.

Used for nervous excitement, dizzyness, headaches and sleeplessness in children, mixed with a little water.

Cowslip Ointment
Cowslip ointment is used to clear the complexion and for sunburn, spots and wrinkles. For the recipe, see the one for marigold ointment on p. 35, substituting cowslip for marigold.

Cowslip Mead
To every 3½ litres (1 gallon) of water add 1 kg (2 lb) of honey and boil for three to four hours. Skim well. Remove 600 ml (1 pint) of the liquid, slice into it one lemon and set aside. Pour the other liquid into an earthenware bowl and add to it 450 g (1 lb) of cowslip heads. Stir well and cover, keeping in a warm place for twenty-four hours. Stir in the lemon liquid, 2 sprigs of sweet briar and 10 g (1¼ oz) yeast dissolved in a little honey.

Allow the mixture to work for four days. Strain and cork. Keep for six months and then bottle.

Emotional uses
On the emotional plane, cowslip is useful for all blocks to progress: general 'stuckness'; feelings of darkness and hopelessness, of being in a negative state. Cowslip's lightness and yellowness helps to lift the spirits, to open and

expand the heart, to help the spirits rise a little. Use for depression, especially after the death of a loved one, for the feelings of abandonment and desolation, or after the break-up of a relationship and the death of that close connection. Cowslip is used not so much for the acute pain of bereavement but rather for the depression and disillusionment that follows this. It works to try and encourage the yellow light of the heart out from the heart chakra and to push the blue light of the head down the body to the feet and ground it into the earth. For these times it would be good to drink warmed cowslip wine or a sweetened tisane. But in the case of deep depression or after a death, make a taliswomyn, wear it and sleep with it around the pillow to banish sorrow and the rage of the bereaved and to allow the trapped energy to be released.

Magical and ritual uses
Cowslip flowers, fresh or dried, were traditionally woven into funeral wreaths which were put on the deceased one's grave each full moon after his or her death. This ritual veneration of the dead was carried on for thirteen moons (one year) afterwards. Posies of cowslip flowers were placed under the pillow before sleeping, if the said person wished to contact the spirit of the recently deceased. Sometimes cowslip flowers were pinned to clothes as a sign of recent bereavement. Sickly babies had cowslip pinned to their cribs to keep away the spirits of the dead.

Love Potion
Cowslip petals were one ingredient of a love potion much used by saxon women. The petals were collected early one morning before the dew had dried on them and put in a container with some fresh rainwater and left all day in sunlight. Then rose petals and violet leaves were added and steeped a further day. A spell was said over the vessel after the second day:

come petals do your best / make me my comliest
so my heart's desire I might obtain
let .... be my swain

The liquid is then collected and sprinkled over the pillow of the beloved. The effects should be seen after a moon (month) has passed. This spell is best done in the first quarter of a moon's cycle.

ELDERFLOWER

Planetary ruler:
Venus

Qualities: *Hot and dry*

Harvest time: *May
and June*

Parts used: *Flowers
and leaves*

Scientific name: *Sambucus
nigra*

Medicinal uses: *For the ear,
nose and throat*

Main constituents: *tannis,
flavonoids, including rutin,
mucilage, essential oil.*

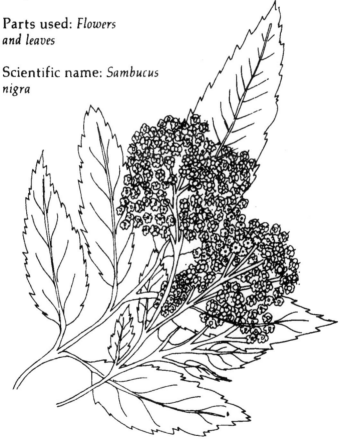

Myths and legends
Elder was one of the sacred trees of the Celts. She was Ruis the Elder, the tree of the thirteenth month. Each of the thirteen lunar months had a tree ascribed to it. (see p. xi)

An instrument called the sambuca was made from the wood of the elder and played in mediaeval and renaissance times.

In Denmark, the elder tree mother, Hylde Moer, a dryad (wood nymph), lived in the elder tree and watched over it. She would haunt anyone who cut her wood without permission as this had to be granted before a single branch was cut. She would give her consent by keeping silence.

The wood-cutter would say:

Lady Ellhorn give me some of thy wood
I will give some of mine when it grows in the forest.

Also in Denmark, it was believed that if you stood under an elder tree on Midsummer Eve you would see the queen of the faeries ride by with all her retinue.

In an English tradition, elderleaves were gathered on May Eve and fixed to doors and windows to keep away witches. Elder twigs were also fastened to cattle sheds to keep evil away from animals.

Russian folk tales also speak of elder blossoms driving away evil spirits, and Sicilians think the tree will kill serpents and keep away robbers. Serbs traditionally used elder blossom in their wedding ceremonies as it was believed to bring good luck. Gypsies will never burn an elder tree for fear of the demons it might release.

Cradles should never be made of elderwood; tradition has it that a child was once put in such a cradle and the *Hylde Moer* came and pulled it by the legs and would give it no peace until it was lifted out.

The tree has a narcotic smell and nobody every slept underneath it. It was believed that visions of fairyland might be seen in such a drugged sleep. Indeed, no plant will grow under the shadow of the tree and this gives weight to the tradition.

Physical uses

This remedy is specific for phlegm, especially in the head. Therefore it can be used with great effect for colds, catarrh, sinus problems, tonsilitis, chronic sore throats and any excess secretion of mucus from head or lungs. It influences the fluid balance in the body, and can be used for water retention, excessive bruising and general sluggishness. It is excellent for those children who seem to have perpetual runny noses, or coughs, colds and adenoid problems. Often excess mucous is due to a reaction to dairy produce (also ruled by Venus). It is a good idea to give such children a dairy-free diet for a month to see if this alleviates their catarrh problems.

Elderflower is a sedative and can be drunk as a tea before sleeping. It can be used to treat disturbed sleep and nightmares.

The herb increases the production of sweat and can be used in feverish colds and flu to help lower the temperature, taken hot as a tea. As a diaphoretic (sweat-inducing) remedy, elderflower is also excellent for the skin; it helps to clear the pores and clear up pimples and acne.

Juliette Bairacli de Levy, in her book *The Illustrated Herbal Handbook*, claims that when blindness is the result of shocks and blasts or nerve damage, elderflowers can help to restore damaged sight (p. 7).

Recipes

Elderflower Champagne

4 heads of elderflower
750 g (1½ lb) of sugar
2 x 15 ml (2 tbsp) white wine vinegar
3½ litres (1 gallon) cold water
2 lemons

Put elderflowers, sugar, vinegar and water into a bowl. Squeeze the lemons and add the juice to the mixture. Cut the lemon skins in quarters and add to the liquid. Leave to stand for twenty-four hours, stirring occasionally. Strain and bottle in screw-topped bottles.

The mixture will be ready to drink in a few days.

Elderflower Poultice
Take equal quantities of elderflower and honeysuckle flowers and add enough water to barely cover and cook until softened. Cool and soak a cloth in the mixture and apply to any hot and painful area.

Elderflower Ointment

225 g (8 oz) elder leaves
100 g (4 oz) plantain leaves
50 g (2 oz) ground ivy
100 g (4 oz) wormwood

Melt 1.75 kg (4 lb) solid vegetable fat or 2 litres (3½ pints) vegetable oil with 50 g (2 oz) beeswax. Simmer the herbs in this for three to four hours; allow to cool and store in a cool place.

For softening hard swellings and wounds.

Elderflower Water (Aqua Sambuci)
Fill a large earthenware jar with the flowers and pour on three pints of boiling water. Allow to cool and add 40 g (1½ oz) of rectified spirits (that is, ethyl alcohol, which can be bought in a chemist). Cover and stand for a few hours, then strain and bottle. Use as a skin lotion for sunburn, blemishes and pimples. This mixture acts as a mild astringent.

Elderberry Syrup
To each gallon of elderberries, add 15 g (½ oz) whole ginger and 18 cloves. Add enough water to prevent burning and boil for one hour and then strain. To every pint of liquid, use 1 kg (2 lb) of fine sugar. Gently melt the sugar in the liquid until there are no grains left, then cool and bottle.

Take 1 x 5 ml (teaspoon) daily during the winter months in warm water.

Mixture for feverish colds and flu
Take equal parts of mint, yarrow and elderflowers and half of fresh ground ginger. Put in a saucepan with cold water, bring to the boil, turn off the heat and keep covered for twenty minutes. Strain and take 1 wineglass full every three hours for up to five days.

Emotional uses
Elder has had a long association with death and bewitchment. It is a light, airy, expansive plant, useful to lighten heavy, stuck, congested emotional states. It gladdens the heart and opens out and lifts the spirits upwards. It can be used to allay nightmares and the night terrors of children. Use for those who find life a struggle or dying people who cannot let go of life because of fear. It eases the passing, the transition to death. It is for people who worry to ease the cloud of confusion and to help them move above their problems and gain some perspective. There is, too, a sense of innocence about the plant. It is for those who have become cynical about life and who have lost their innocence and have become hard. It may be used after loss, hard times and long illnesses, to connect with hope.

Sleep with a bunch of dried flowers under your pillow. If you wish, place these in a cotton bag.

Magical and ritual uses
Elder wood traditionally is used to make wands. They are as long as the distance between your armpit and the end of your middle finger. Take the wood at the time of the full moon and pay for it with a drop of your own blood. Hollow out one end, push in a piece of cloth coated with a drop of your menstrual blood and seal with candlewax.

The name of the witch was carved on to the wand in the local language or in the magical language of the runes. Traditionally, wands were made at the time of the fire new moon (Aries, Leo, Saggitarius). Wands were passed three times through the flames of a ritual fire and annointed with special oils.

Beltane ritual

Beltane (30 April) was the time when young women who had had their first menstruation, were initiated into women's mysteries. All the participants wore garlands of spring flowers and crowns woven from elder and may blossoms. Elder, and hawthorn (may) represented the planets Venus and Mars, or male and female energies. This was the time of the first coming together of young men and women. Brigid, the fairy queen, presided over the festivities; she was invoked by the Goddess whose origins are lost in the mists of antiquity.

Hear the words of the star goddess, the dust of whose feet are the hosts of heaven,
Whose body encircles the universe
I who am the beauty of the green earth and the white moon among the stars
and the mysteries of the waters,
I call upon your soul to arise and come unto Me.
For I am the soul of nature that gives life to the universe.
From Me all things proceed and unto Me they must return
Let My worship be in the heart that rejoices, for behold,
all acts of love and pleasure are My rituals.
Let there be beauty and strength, power and compassion,
honour and humility
mirth and reverence within you.
And you seek to know Me, know that your seeking and yearning will avail
you not, unless you know the mystery:
for if that which you seek, you find not within yourself,
you will never find it without.
For behold, I have been with you from the beginning, and am that which is attained at the end of desire.

(From *The Spiral Dance*, by Starhawk, p. 76.)

Silence follows in order to meditate on these words. A toast is then made to the goddess of May. Ritual singing and dancing follow. The circle is closed and women celebrate.

LADY'S MANTLE

Planetary ruler: *Venus*

Qualities: *Hot and dry*

Harvest time: *June and July*

Plants used: *Flowers and leaves*

Scientific name: *Alchemilla vulgaris*

Medicinal uses: *For gynaecological conditions
and obstetrics*

Main constituents: *Tannins, bitters,
salicylic acid.*

Myths and legends

The name *Alchemilla* is said to have come from the Arabic *Alkmelych*, meaning alchemy.

The plant was believed to possess magical powers and was used by the alchemists in their experiments. The dew which formed on the leaves of lady's mantle was collected on summer mornings and was believed to have had many mystical qualities. The Arabs thought alchemy was invented by the Egyptians and the Christians learnt it from the Arabs.

Mary the Jewess was said to have been the first great alchemist, according to Carl Jung in *Man and His Symbols* (p. 186). She invented the distillation of alcohol and the double boiler, or *bain marie*. During the Renaissance, female alchemists were burned as witches; the Duke of Brunswick roasted one alive in a chair in 1575 because she would not tell him how to turn base metal into gold.

Alchemists sought the devine female power *Sapientia* or Sophia – (wisdom) – the great mother of the gnostics. The philosphical stone was sometimes called the sophistical stone. The great mother was shown by the holy vase. Alchemists sought the *vas hermeticum* (womb of Hermes).

I am the flower of the field and the lily of the valleys.
I am the mother of fair love and of fear and of knowledge
   and of holy hope.
I am the mediator of the elements
I am the law in the priest and the word in the prophet and
   the counsel in the wise.
I will kill and I will make to live and there is none that can
   deliver out of my hand.

Hermes was the alchemist hero who fertilised the holy vase, or womb, from which the *filius philosorum* (the son of the philosophers) was born. The menstrual blood of the Great Whore, a name for the Great Mother, was said to have curdled in her womb to create the universe, including its metals, minerals and other raw materials of alchemy.

Physical uses
This is the principle herb used for gynaecological conditions, the first herb of choice for all problems and imbalances affecting the womb and ovaries. With painful periods, it clears up cramps after one to two months' use. I have had wonderful results using this herb with women who are getting older (that is, over 35) and trying to conceive for the first time. It is usually effective two months after taking the herb. I also give lady's mantle to pregnant women who fear miscarriage and who are having a lot of pain, or who are losing small amounts of blood. It helps to prepare for labour but, as it is such a strong astringent, it is best used for women who have had many children and perhaps lack muscle tone, or those women with weakened cervices who have had miscarriages and abortions. Astringents dry up secretions, so lady's mantle can be used to reduce the amount of blood loss in a period and to curb post-partum bleeding, that is, heavier than normal blood loss in the days after childbirth. After delivery its use will help the uterus to regain its natural size and it is also helpful where there is a possibility of prolapse. It also helps the breasts to regain their elasticity. As a general tonic to the reproductive

system, lady's mantle can be used where there has been physical trauma to the area, such as abortion, miscarriage, IUD insertion/extraction, thrush, pelvic inflammatory disease or fibroids. It can also be used for heavy bleeding at the menopause and to reduce the excess sweating which sometimes occurs at this time. It is a wound healer and can be used both internally as a tea or tincture or externally as a lotion, as in episiotomies, for example.

Lady's mantle is a prime example of a herb of Venus acting in sympathy with nature to build up weakened tissue and strengthen the organs she rules.

Recipes

To increase fertility

Mix together a tincture of lady's mantle and vitex.

Take 20 drops first thing in the morning for up to six months.

For healing the womb after trauma (such as rape, abortion, surgery)

10 g (¼ oz) lady's mantle
10 g (¼ oz) mugwort

Make a tea of the above ingredients.

Take for at least one menstrual cycle and for up to three months.

WARNING. Not to be taken in pregnancy.

Emotional uses

Alchemilla is an especially useful herb for earth-bound people who are stuck in mundane reality and wish to connect with different realms but cannot make the transition. Being an alchemic plant, lady's mantle can help people to make life changes when they are afraid to take the risk. It is a herb for breaking umbilical ties, for moving away from the past. It works on the brow chakra to give clarity and clear vision. It is strengthening and helps women prepare for acts of courage, for the way of the warrior, or for trials of strength and endurance, such as mountain climbing, exams, childbirth and initiation rites. Give to women who may be holding back from labour through fear.

Put 15 ml (1 tablespoon) of dried flowers in a cotton bag and place in a bath of hot water. Lie in this for ten to fifteen minutes.

Because of its association with the warrior, use lady's mantle for any death, trauma, pain and despair over childbirth; for times when death is a whisper away. On a deeper level, there is a connection with the rage and despair that is woman, to the primal scream of fury and anguish at the cruelty, pain and suffering in the world. The herb is for any women who has suffered at the hands of patriarchy, been cruelly treated or tortured.

Lady's mantle also operates on the womb chakra and is therefore connected with creativity. It is for women who are blocked creatively and to lighten up the emotional charge behind the creative act, allowing the creativity to flow more freely, to flourish.

Sprinkle the powdered dried herb on a disc of charcoal each night and take some time to sit and contemplate the acts of creation you wish to perform.

Allow yourself to dream a little. Imagine how it will be to be more creative; how it will feel, how it will change your life, your relationships, your feeling about yourself. This need only take ten minutes daily. Record your thoughts in a diary and from time to time read through your entries to see the progress you have made.

Magical and ritual uses

Conception ritual

There are believed to be two times in her monthly cycle when a woman is fertile. The first is when the moon is at the same phase as when the woman was born (that is, as found in her natal chart) and the second twelve to fourteen days after her last period started. Here is a ritual which can be performed by women wanting to conceive:

At your fertile time (but never at the full moon, because it is said children conceived at this time will be born crazy – lunatics), light a white candle and draw down into your body the moon's rays. Feel the silvery light flood your whole being, from your head to your feet. Bathe in her fecund energies and be aware of any images or thoughts which come to mind. Allow a symbol to emerge for your fertility. Concentrate on the symbol, feel it becoming alive and potent. Invoke the goddess of fertility, the mother aspect of the Triple Goddess, and say the words:

> *Mother I call you now,*
> *Come, come and bring the spirit of my child with you*
> *I want a child.*
> *Grant me my wish.*
> *She will be a child of the Goddess*
> *Wise in the Old Ways*[1]

This ritual takes two months in all. At the first month, just after the last bleed, go on a short, cleansing fast. Eat raw fruit and vegetables, organic ones if possible. Drink lots of spring water to cleanse the system. During the two-month period, try not to take any wine or stimulants of any kind. Drink a cup of lady's mantle both morning and evening. At ovulation, about fourteen days later, perform the first half of the ritual and then, when the moon is new, the second half. All that time drink lady's mantle twice daily and you will conceive at the next fertile time.

MUGWORT

Planetary ruler: *Venus*

Qualities: *Hot and dry*

Harvest time: *June to August*

Parts used: *Flowers and leaves*

Scientific name: *Artemisia vulgaris*

Medicinal uses: *For gynaecological symptoms and the blood*

Main constituents: *Volatile oil (thujone), tannins, bitters.*

Myths and legends

Mugwort was one of the nine sacred herbs from the *Lacnunga*, a Saxon text on herbal medicine:

> *eldest of worts*
> *thou hast might for three*
> *and against thirty*
> *for venom availest*
> *for flying vile things*
> *might against loathed ones*
> *that through the land rove.*

The Latin name, *artemisia*, refers to the goddess Artemis who was the symbol of herbal practitioners in many countries. Artemis was the Amazon moon goddess; she was mother of all creatures. She was shown in images as a figure with a thousand breasts. Iphigenia, the priestess of Artemis, sacrificed all men who landed on Tauris, the island where she lived, nailing the head of each to a wooden cross. In Attica the goddess was worshipped with drops of blood from the necks of men, symbolic of the ancient beheadings.

Thousand-breasted Artemis was the patron and protector of all animals, of fertility and birth. She was also represented by the great she-bear, Ursa major, ruler of the stars and protector of the *axis mundi* (pole of the world) marked by the pole star at the centre of the constellation of Ursa major.

Ephesus was the shrine of Artemis, founded by the amazons, built around the holy tree.

In mediaeval England, mugwort was associated with witchcraft and a bunch of it was hung on the inside of a doorway to keep evil away and to protect the house from lightning.

Pliny in his *Natural History* reported that a traveller wearing mugwort would not suffer from weariness and would not be hurt by poison or wild beasts.[2]

Physical uses

Mugwort acts as a relaxant and astringent and is especially useful for girls at puberty when periods can be very painful and bleeding excessively long and heavy. By its heat, mugwort dries up excessive blood and thus reduces menstrual loss. It helps to regulate the menstrual cycle, bringing it more in line with the lunar cycle. Taken hot, it will help to bring on a delayed period. It is a powerful blood cleanser and can be used as a European alternative to echinacea, an antiseptic remedy from the USA, for any strong infection or infestation. As a bitter, mugwort stimulates the action of the liver which explains its blood cleansing action. It is also used as a digestive stimulant, for nausea, appetite loss and as a general tonic to stimulate the metabolism and the excretion of wastes from the body. It is unwise to take during pregnancy. As an antiseptic, use mugwort in a tea or tincture for pelvic inflammatory disease, chronic thrush or cystitis, or any womb infection. It can be used concurrently with antibiotics for venereal diseases and will help to minimise the suppressant effect of these drugs.

Recipes

In Cornwall, at the turn of the century, dried mugwort leaves were used as a substitute for tea which was too expensive for ordinary people.

To bring on a delayed period

Use equal parts (eg 20 g (⅓ oz) each of mugwort, southernwood and pennyroyal.
Add 600 ml (1 pint) boiling water. Cover and stand for twenty minutes.
Drink in the course of a day.

For infertility (from Trotula)

15 g (½ oz) mallow
15 g (½ oz) mugwort
600 ml (1 pint) water

Make a tea and strain.
Use 1 cup of the mixture to douche twice a week to strengthen the vaginal area.

For bleeding after delivery (after Trotula)

Mix 5 g (⅛ oz) each of mugwort, sage and pennyroyal with water. Sip warm as a tea.

Emotional uses

I associate mugwort with the brow chakra, the third eye, which gives us our clairvoyant powers and the ability to see clearly, and also with the throat chakra, the ability to be creative and self-expressive. It allows a woman to connect with her own source of strength and power, her own inner resources; it is affirming, stabilising and strengthening. It helps to unblock ambition and allow for the leader within to emerge.
When you need clarity and strength, make a tea of mugwort and drink before going to bed at night.

Magical and ritual use

The psychic and ritual uses of mugwort are legion. I have included those which seem appropriate in the context of this book, but be aware that there are many many more.

Incense - for fertility of both womb and ideas

Mix together: myrrh crystals, frankincense, sandlewood oil, mugwort, yarrow and juniper berries. Steep in spirit or wine for at least two weeks. Strain out and allow to dry gently, say, next to a fire or on a radiator. Store in a screw-topped jar.

Use when the Moon is full and in an Earth sign, or Libra.

Burn a little mugwort on a charcoal disc and meditate on your blocks to creativity. Think of the creative acts you wish to perform and allow the images of these acts to become clear. Imagine yourself doing these things; allow your vision to become real to you. On black paper write with a silver pen your image of your next creative move. Tie the paper up with red thread and, dedicating your work to Artemis, burn the paper in a candle flame imaging the seeds of your vision scattering in your world and taking root and growing there.

A taliswomyn for travellers and lovers of the night

On a waning moon, preferably when it is in Virgo, mix together yarrow, mugwort, fleabane, cat's paw and lady's finger in equal parts. Add sandlewood oil and oil of myrrh. Steep in a little spirit or wine for one whole moon.

Dry out and dedicate on your altar to Hecate, goddess of the night, and travellers in wild places. Add to the mixture some juniper berries and comfrey bells and sew the mixture into a black or silver bag. Tie this up with a red cord. Knot the cord thirteen times, saying:

> Lady of the nightime terrors
> of dark and windy places,
> as I carry this tailswomyn on my journeys,
> protect me from all fears and dangers.

> *Lady of the darkness heal and protect me,*
> *so mote it be.*

Wear this when you travel or when you feel fearful of darkness. Renew each year after the full moon in Virgo.

To consecrate a magical object

At the full moon, boil up a handful of mugwort (fresh or dried) with yarrow and some sandlewood. When it has come to the boil, turn off the heat and let it stand, covered, for thirty minutes. Dip a white cloth into the mixture and carefully wash the object to be purified, while saying the following words:

> *Moon, Moon, wash away*
> *wash away*
> *all impurities*
> *all bad energies*
> *fill this . . . . . . with light*
> *with love,*
> *with wisdom,*
> *So mote it be,*
> *Blessed Be.*

Hold the object up into the light of the full moon and feel its power being absorbed. Feel the object fill with the power of the Goddess. Wrap it in black silk to contain its energy and keep in a sacred space.

Use for crystal balls, tarot cards, crystals and magic mirrors.

For dreams, scrying and astral travel

Mugwort works on the brow chakra. Before doing any such work, drink a strong brew of mugwort and/or put it in your ritual bathwater. It will allow you to travel further, to see more clearly and to do magic work in your dream life.

Dreams can be used to work magically. The images and symbols which arise in dreams have a powerful effect on the psyche. It is possible to ask for a dream before falling asleep which will clarify a problem or shed light on a conflict or difficulty you have in your life. The more attention you pay to your dreams, the more vivid they become. Keep a notebook by the side of your bed to record them immediately on waking. Dreams sometimes come in sequences as a major difficulty is gradually resolved.

It is possible to have a dialogue with different characters or objects in your dream. Find a quiet spot where you will be undisturbed for at least half an hour. Sit in a comfortable position and take a few deep breaths to relax and calm yourself. Close your eyes and recall your dream, allowing the images to become vivid. Choose one character, or it may be an object such as a house, the sea or an animal. Become that person or object. Then allow it to speak freely, without trying to analyse what it says. You may then want to move on to another character or object. Repeat the process. If it feels appropriate, allow the different parts of the dream to have a dialogue. This does not have to be done all at once; an important dream may need several sessions for its meaning to become clear.

To develop psychic skills (scrying), power objects such as crystal balls or tarot cards can be used for gaining information or clarity about an issue.

Find a quiet spot where you will be undisturbed for at least half an hour. Sit in a comfortable position with your spine straight. Take a few deep breaths to relax and centre yourself. Hold the ball at least 46 centimetres (18 inches) away from your gaze. Don't stare. You need to half-close your eyes, to put them almost out of focus. Remembering to breathe and trying to keep relaxed, allow yourself to become receptive to whatever will appear. To begin with, you will see nothing, but gradually the ball will become cloudy and then through the cloud images will begin to appear. Don't do this for too long to begin with, as it can be really tiring. Also, the work is not easy to do and, like any other skill, it needs practice and determination to accomplish.

When we sleep, we leave our physical bodies and enter the astral plane. Anyone who has ever been woken suddenly from sleep will know that this causes a shock or jolt to the system. This is because you have to return very rapidly from the astral plane to this world. With practice, this can be achieved not only when sleeping but at will. The most common fear of someone who is astral travelling is that she will not return, or that she will get lost somewhere in the astral plane. I have never heard of this happening, but for reassurance do astral travel work with a friend. Ask her to sit by you so that you can reach out and touch her should you feel afraid.

Lie down in a comfortable spot. Take several deep breaths to relax the mind and body. Allow your attention to focus on the centre of your body. Feel yourself becoming smaller and smaller until you are tiny. Then imagine yourself becoming bigger again until you are enormous and fill up the room you are in. Return to normal size and imagine yourself floating above your body. See your body lying on the floor and become aware of a golden thread connecting your floating self with the body on the floor. This is your connection; at any time you can return to your body by following the cord back to its source. (The cord cannot break or be severed in any way.)

Allow yourself to float up through the ceiling, through the roof of your house and over the place where you live. Moving further and further up, see the land slowly moving away from you as you travel further and further into space. When you are in space, look around for a guide. This may appear in the form of a person, a symbol or an object. Allow the guide to take you where it wants. You will be led to a place where work needs to be done or where you will meet others travelling in a similar fashion. Spend time there. Then, when you feel ready, slowly repeat what you have done in reverse, allowing yourself to come gently back down again to earth, to your house and finally to your body. When you are back, take time to feel focused in your physical body. Twitch your toes, move your hands and feet, and then slowly sit up. Write down your experience immediately, to remember it, and be clear about the details. Afterwards, talk over what happened with your friend.

PENNYROYAL

Planetary ruler: *Venus*

Qualities:
Hot and dry

Harvest time:
August

Parts used:
Flowers and leaves

Scientific name:
Mentha pulegium

Medicinal uses: *For*
gynaecological conditions

Main constituents:
volatile oil, tannins

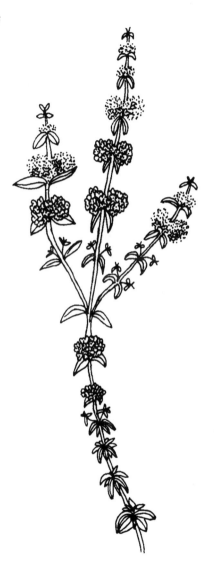

Myths and legends
Pennyroyal was called 'pudding grass' as it was used to stuff hogs' puddings. A famous stuffing used to be made of pennyroyal, honey and pepper.

It was said that if you tied pennyroyal to the bedpost it would increase the power of the brain and make that person more alert and aware.

Traditionally it was carried by seafarers to prevent sea sickness.

Physical action
Being hot and dry, pennyroyal opposes the natural function of the womb in that it expels accumulated matter within it, acting by antipathy. Traditionally used as an abortive herb, it works powerfully and can cause acute stomach cramps in the process. **For this reason it is *never* to be used by pregnant women as it will cause a miscarriage and certainly damage the foetus.** It has a distinctive smell which all kinds of flies and insects, mosquitoes and midges, find most unappealing; an oil can be made of the herb and rubbed on the body to keep away persistent pests. It will also bannish fleas and other creepy crawlies. As it is a hot herb, it can be used for menstrual cramps induced by the cold to heat up the womb and allow for the free flowing of the menstrual blood. It can help to strengthen the mother exhausted after childbirth. The volatile oil is a strong antiseptic and pennyroyal can be used locally for infected gums, sore throats or septic wounds.

Pennyroyal is a powerful blood cleanser and, as a herb of Venus, clears the lungs of thick phlegm. It is also a traditional remedy for dizzyness and pains in the head.

Recipes
Expectorant (after Culpeper)

25 g (1 oz) pennyroyal
5 ml (1 teasp) honey
5 ml (1 teasp) salt
600 ml (1 pint) water

Mix the pennyroyal, honey and salt together. Add the water and simmer for a while. Strain.

Drink this to expel thick phlegm from the lungs.

To facilitate childbirth (after Trotula)

    5 ml (1 teasp) dried mint
    5 ml (1 teasp) dried pennyroyal
    5 ml (1 teasp) dried marjoram

Mix together.

Place on a piece of charcoal to burn as an incense and sit above the steaming bowl. (Presumably this stimulates the contractions and dilation of the cervix.)

Emotional uses

Pennyroyal works on the womb centre and helps to focus a woman's energy to make her aware of her own root power, to help her to be less susceptible to the will of others, to stop her being confused by too many people's opinions and to help her stop feeling the victim of what others do to her. It is for those who feel attacked by the ill-will of others. It rebuilds the centre of a woman, after serious illness or too many children, when she feels she has lost the thread of her own identity and needs to rebuild the web of her own centre of power.

Add 1 drop of the essential oil to your bathwater, or 15 ml (1 tablespoonful) of the dried herb if the oil is unobtainable.

WARNING. Do not use if you are pregnant.

Magical and ritual uses
A spell to stop a run of bad luck

At the New Moon make an incense of the following finely ground herbs: pennyroyal, sage, frankincense and sandlewood. Bind the mixture together with honey and brandy and leave out to dry. Set up an altar with three white candles and one black and one orange candle. Light the incense. The three white candles represent your body, feelings and mind, the black candle all the bad luck you have had, while the orange candle is the good luck which will come to you.

Light the white candles one by one, saying:

May my body have health and strength
may my feelings be calm and serene
may my mind think clearly and wisely.

Light the black candle, saying:

May all my bad luck leave with the flames of this candle.

Light the orange, saying:

May good luck come to me,
so mote it be.

Meditate on how you want your life to be, what changes need to happen. Try to be as specific and as clear as possible. The better you can visualise what you want the more likely it is that it will come to pass. Affirm to yourself that within one month life will have changed.

THYME

Planetary ruler: *Venus*

Qualities: *Hot and dry*

Harvest time: *June to September*

Parts used: *Flowers and leaves*

Scientific name: *Thymus vulgaris*

Medicinal uses: *For the lungs and
as an antiseptic*

Main constituents: *volatile oil, which contains
thymol, bitters, tannins,
flavonoids, triterpenoids.*

Myths and legends

Thymus comes from the Greek *thumus*, meaning courage, and also 'to fumigate'. It was a great invigorating herb and was used to inspire courage.

Thyme used to be used as a fumigator to keep pests away from the home.

Among the Greeks, the smell of thyme was an expression of praise for those who were fashionable. It was a symbol of activity, bravery and courage.

In the age of chivalry, women used to embroider handkerchiefs showing a bee hovering over a sprig of thyme to give to their knights.

In the south of France, thyme was a symbol of republicanism, sprigs of thyme being sent as a message for meetings.

Physical uses

Thyme is an antiseptic remedy and can be used wherever there is infection. In my experience it works particularly well for lung and kidney infections, but can be used safely for anywhere in the body. Thyme is a strong remedy and is best taken in short, sharp doses that is, from seven to ten days only at a time. I *never* give it to anyone for longer than three consecutive weeks. If the infection has not cleared up by then, there are probably other factors which have not been addressed. Use it therefore for bronchitis, tonsilitis, pleurisy, septic sore throats, ear infections and whooping cough. It is also the remedy of choice for cystitis, combined with bearberry. If taken, it will clear up the infection in three to four days with no need for antibiotics. Thyme also helps to expel mucous from the lungs and therefore can be used for dry, irritating coughs. It purges the body of phlegm and regulates the humoural balance of phelgm in the body, riding it of excess. It is also a diaphoretic (sweat-inducing) remedy and so can be used to great effect for colds and flu where you need to lower the temperature and cleanse the body quickly. Thyme is also slightly sedative and so can be used for nervous headaches and insomnia. It can be used in a bath to alleviate the pains of rheumatism and also as a lotion for itchy skin, hives and ringworm. It is said to help with childbirth and with the delivery of the placenta which fits well with its planetary rulership.

Recipes
For Cystitis and urethritis (inflammation of the urethra)

25 g (1 oz) thyme
25 g (1 oz) bearberry

Add 1.2 litres (2 pints) of boiling water.
Drink warm during the course of the day. Repeat for three days until the symptoms have gone.

Syrup of Thyme for whooping cough

225 g (8 oz) thyme
900 ml (1½ pints) of spring water

Pour the boiling water over the flowers placed in a saucepan, and close the vessel.
Let stand in a warm place such as a slow-cooker, Rayburn or

radiator for twelve hours. Strain and measure the liquid. To every pint, add 1 kg (2 lb) caster sugar, melted and scummed. Stir over a low heat until it is well mixed.

Dose: 1 x 5 ml (tea)spoon every three hours.

Cough Lozenges

15 g (½ oz) thyme
15 g (½ oz) fennel
15 g (½ oz) coltsfoot

Add to 3 cups of boiling water and infuse overnight. Strain and add 1 cup of set honey or maple syrup and simmer until the mixture begins to thicken. Pour on to an oiled backing sheet and cut into squares as it cools.

Dose: Not more than five lozenges daily, to be taken for ten days.

Emotional uses

Thyme has the quality of an eagle, soaring high amongst mountain peaks in the half light before dawn when it is darkest, coldest and quietest. It is for those who have suffered much, who feel they have come to the end of their strength and have reached their lowest point, when all seems lost, futile and hopeless but also where there is the feeling that this feeling too shall pass, a timeless unreal quality that life sometimes has. The herb is for when it seems as if the pulse of life has stopped beating – it is so still. Thyme gives strength and courage to hold on until things improve. It allows a woman to make the step from darkness to light, from death to life, from the unreal to the real, to have the faith to keep on, although weakness and exhaustion are great. It is for major life traumas – deaths, births, separations and tragedies – to give a woman the stamina to see everything through and to emerge as if reborn into the daylight.

Burn dried thyme on charcoal each night before sleeping.

Ask for dreams to help you. Do this for as long as you feel
the need.

Magical and ritual uses
Ritual to banish fear and inspire courage
Choose a full Moon of water (that is Pisces, Cancer or,
preferably, Scorpio); take yourself to a sacred space and
make a circle, invoking the four elements. To do this, walk
slowly and purposefully in a circle in an anti-clockwise
direction. As you walk the circle, sprinkle dried thyme to
mark its boundaries. Invoke Diana the Huntress, leader of
the amazon warriors, and bid her give you courage in this
ritual. Sit in the centre of the circle and have incense
burning which has thyme as one of its ingredients. Visualise
one of your greatest fears; take time to do this. Imagine
your fear in all its aspects, its terrifying nature and how it
manifests (or might manifest) in your everyday life. As you
do this, be aware of your body, make sure you keep
breathing and notice where in your body this fear is located,
how you physically feel this fear. Then become aware of
your breathing; see how you take your breaths and
gradually lengthen your inhalations and exhalations, still
holding the image of your fear clear in your mind. Direct
your breath to that place where you feel the fear and allow
yourself to breathe into that place. Continue this for a
while and then breathe white light into this place, healing,
protective white light. Continue and then allow this white
light to fill your whole body, protecting you and banishing
your fear.

Now look at your fear from the centre of this light. See
what has changed about it, how it looks to you now. Take
some time to do this, observing this fear now you are
surrounded and protected by white light. See if anything
has changed, what looks different now. In your imagination,
act as if you were no longer afraid of this thing, that you
have courage. How would it look? What would you be doing
if you had courage? How does it feel to act in this way, to
have courage? Take some time to explore your world now

you have courage! See how your everyday world might change. Be aware of your body as you do this: how does it feel, what is different? Finally, let this image go and stand in the centre of your circle, and without 'thinking of it' take on a posture which embodies the courage you have just experienced. Experiment, and when you have found the right posture, stand in it and really allow yourself to feel courageous; feel yourself filled with white light and protected from any danger. Take some time to assimilate this experience, sitting quietly.

When you feel ready, thank the Goddess for her presence and inspiration and unwind the circle. To do this, slowly and purposefully walk in a circle, moving in a clockwise direction. Thank the four elements and leave the place.

During the next moon cycle, take time to practise this. Adopt the posture whenever you feel afraid. Surround yourself with white light and act as if you had courage.

VERVAIN

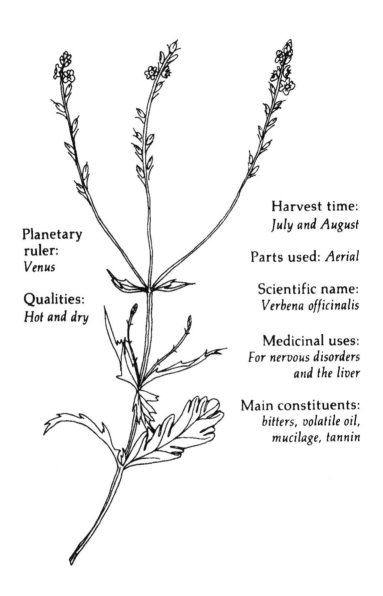

Planetary
ruler:
Venus

Qualities:
Hot and dry

Harvest time:
July and August

Parts used: *Aerial*

Scientific name:
Verbena officinalis

Medicinal uses:
*For nervous disorders
and the liver*

Main constituents:
*bitters, volatile oil,
mucilage, tannin*

Myths and legends

Vervain comes from the Celtic word *ferfaen, fer* meaning to drive away and *faen* a stone.

Vervain was used by the druids as an ingredient in their lustral water, a secret and magical fluid, and for spells, incantations and divination. The plant was prepared by steeping it in cold water and then infusing it in wine and boiling it. It was used in ointments, fumigation salves and magic medicine. It was also used as an amulet for protection. The druid ritual when collecting vervain stated it should be picked when the Moon was dark and the dog star had just risen. In the place where the herb was picked, a honeycomb was left as restitution for the violence done to the earth.

Vervain may have been introduced to Rome by the druids; it was certainly used by the Romans as a ritual cleansing plant, and called Britannica. It was made into bundles which were used as brooms to sweep the altars and dust the table of Jupiter. A festival named Verbenalia was held each July in recognition of the plant. The herb was dedicated to Venus and used in many love potions and carried in posies by the women of Rome.

Vervain was used both to prevent witchcraft being done to a person and as a main ingredient in many spells and potions. It was also said to have an effect on dreams; worn as an amulet or tied above the bed it was said to prevent nightmares and bad dreams.

Vervain was traditionally given to babies to make them learn quickly. In rural areas it was dug into ploughed fields to encourage the growth of crops.

It was said that those who rubbed themselves with vervain oil would attain all they desired.

Vervain was used in times of plague to ward off infection and calamity. The *Grete Herbal* of 1526 (to be found in Queen's College, Oxford), has this recipe:

To make folk merry at table: take 4 leaves and 4 roots of vervain, steep them in wine and then sprinkle about the house where the guests will be.

Vervain was called the herb of grace.

Physical uses

Vervain acts as a powerful remedy for the nervous system. It is deep-acting and takes at least a month to work. Use for all kinds of upsets of the nervous system: anxiety, depression, fearfulness, insomnia, irritability, headaches, general nervous over-sensitivity and weakness. It is an excellent remedy to use for someone who is coming off tranquillisers or other mood-altering drugs; it will help to build up the nervous system's strength and resilience, making the person less reactive to stress.

The herb is an excellent remedy for fear and frenzy. The bitter in vervain accounts for its action on the liver and digestive system in general. It can be used for digestive conditions associated with nervous strain, such as ulcers, colitis and heartburn. It can also be used for more serious liver complaints, such as cirrhosis and jaundice and persistant viral conditions of the liver.

Vervain increases sweat production in the body and therefore can be used for infectious fevers, debilitating fevers such as malaria and summer fever in children. Vervain is also a remedy for the female reproductive system and is used in the long-term treatment of pre-menstrual migraine and painful periods. It also increases the flow of breast milk. Vervain has a slight stimulant action on the womb and for that reason should not be used by pregnant women, although it is fine for breast-feeding mothers. It helps to relieve menstrual cramps caused by the cold and treats sickness in the womb. Vervain is hot, dry and bitter, opening obstruction, cleansing and healing. It cleanses the kidneys and bladder of those sediments which build up into stones, and expels gravel. As an antispasmodic remedy, vervain is useful for all spasms in the body: stomach cramps, palpitations, asthma and whooping cough.

Externally it is used as a mouthwash for dental decay and gum disease, for tonsilitis, sore throats and facial neuralgia.

Vervain is helpful after a debilitating fever and has been

found useful after Myalgic encephalomyelitis (ME) the post-viral syndrome. (Although it is believed to be incurable, the disease can definitely be alleviated with the use of herbs.)

Distilled water of vervain is excellent for the eyes where there are films or cloudiness which affect the eyesight, and it is believed to strengthen the optic nerves.

Recipe
Tea to bring down a fever
Add 1 x 5 ml (tea)spoon of dried and ground vervain to a teacupful of either pennyroyal or raspberry leaf tea.

To be taken every half hour. The patient must be kept warm and also be given a warm tea of ginger root.

Dr Coffin, a nineteenth-century herbalist, states that vervain is the best emetic (vomit-inducing) herb apart from lobelia, and is the strongest sweating mixture. He used it to treat tuberculosis and scurvy and to abort an asthma attack.

WARNING. Any herb which causes vomiting must be used with care as the vomit can be inhaled; this causes choking.

Emotional uses
Vervain works on the solar plexus and throat chakras for those who have experienced an acute trauma, violence, a sudden death or accident, or anything which causes a deep and profound shock to the psyche.

Take 5 drops of the tincture, or a tea if this is not available, during the crisis. Afterwards take a tea every night for as long as you feel the need.

Working on the solar plexus, it helps to seal it and protect the woman from unhelpful influences. On the throat it allows the woman a voice for her grief, the physical release of mourning. After a death, vervain helps to hold the psyche together, preventing fragmentation at this most critical time; it slows the person down, allowing one step to be taken at a time and space for healing and assimilation of the experience, without repression or forcing of the pace. The event may have happened many years previously and only recently have surfaced, as previously the psyche was not strong enough to face the pain.

Generally vervain strengthens, centres and calms the emotions. It will give some degree of balance and objectivity and a measure of solidity to a fragmented or scattered person. It is best avoided by those who are forceful and who tend toward overbearing bossyness, rigidity or emotional dullness, as it may increase their earthiness. Such people have strong opinions and don't change them easily. They try to convert others to their point of view. They often exhaust themselves, pushing beyond their limits. Vervain as a herb of Venus is an excellent remedy for phlegmatics who can get lost in the vast seas of their emotional lives and too easily lose a sense of boundaries and proportion. Vervain's strengthening and focusing qualities can help to put feelings into perspective and allow phlegmatics to cope better with life's emotional ups and downs.

Spell for strength and healing

Use after shock, exhaustion, sickness or grief; whenever a woman needs to tap into and release her inner strengths and vital spirit. To be performed whenever needed, but especially at the full Moon. Set up an altar with one red, one green and one yellow candle. Prepare an incense beforehand of the following finely powdered ingredients: vervain, sage, rosemary and myrrh. Mix with enough honey and brandy to bind them and then leave the mixture to dry. When the first evening star is to be seen, burn the incense and light the candles, one by one. Red is for courage to face the future; green is for love and good health; yellow is for prosperity and plenty.
Then say:

> Goddess, I call on you,
> bring me strength
> Bring me courage
> Bring me wisdom

That I might heal my life and prosper.
Blessed Be

Visualise the next steps you need to take, the hurdles you face. See yourself strong, confident and capable of doing what is needed.

Love potion

    20 g (⅓ oz) elecampagne
    20 g (⅓ oz) vervain
    20 g (⅓ oz) mistletoe

Mix together and dry in a cool oven. Grind into a powder with a pestle and mortar until very fine.

Put a pinch into the wine of your beloved and watch out for the results!

Notes

1. The charge of the Goddess is an ancient invocation. No one knows whence it came or how old it is. It has many versions. See, for instance, Margot Adler, *Drawing Down the Moon*, pp. 57-58. I myself like this poetic version.
2. Pliny, born 23 AD in Como in Italy, wrote his *Natural History* in 77 AD. It comprised thirty-seven volumes, of which seven were devoted to medical botany.

3
HERBS OF THE MOON

Element: *Water*

Organs: *Breasts and stomach*

Realm: *Feeling*

Humour: *Phlegmatic*

Function: *Expulsion*

Qualities: *Cold and moist*

Unlike the herbs of Venus, the herbs of the Moon are far less common. The Moon's quality of coldness and moistness is far stronger than that of Venus and her herbs are more inimical to life. Some of the greatest poisons and narcotics are lunar herbs, such as poppy and henbane. They are poisons because they so chill the body that life cannot be sustained.

Moon herbs are of the phlegmatic humour and, being cold and moist, strengthen the expulsive faculty in the body.

The herbs of the Moon included in this book are chickweed and cleavers.

CHICKWEED

Planetary ruler:
Moon

Qualities: *Cold and moist*

Havest time:
June to August

Parts used: *Aerial*

Scientific name:
Stellaria media

Medical uses: *For the skin and lungs*

Main constituents:
Saponins copper and tin

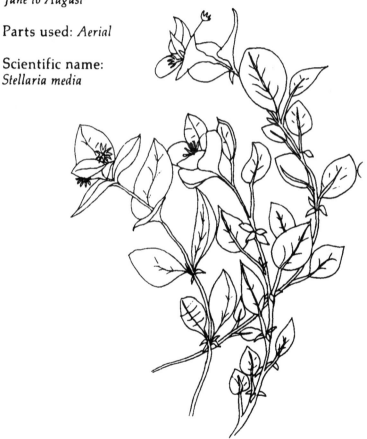

Myths and legends
Other names include satin flower, adder's mouth, starwort, stitchwort and tongue grass.

It is said that there is no part of the world where chickweed cannot be found; it has followed settlers all over temperate regions and the north arctic regions.

The Swiss eat chickweed to strengthen the heart and use it as a convalescent medicine. Traditionally, chickweed has been eaten as a salad vegetable to improve the eyesight, and cooked like spinach to build up the blood.

Physical uses
A cooling remedy for the skin, chickweed is used for eczema, boils, heat rashes, urticaria, (inflammation of the skin) and any hot and irritating skin conditions. Thus it opposes the action of Mars and the Sun, tempering the heat and dryness of these two planets. Chickweed cools the heat of the liver. It is used for inflammation or weakness of the bowels, stomach and lungs, and for any other kind of internal inflammation. It soothes and cools, and is especially useful in colitis and other irritable bowel conditions. Chickweed has an affinity for the lungs and is helpful in cases of bronchitis, pleurisy, coughs, colds and hoarseness. It is used in the treatment of rheumatism, both externally in the form of an ointment and internally.

The herb can be used for blood poisoning and scabies and cleanses the whole system.

A decoction of the fresh plant was used for obesity and cramps.

Use chickweed cream or lotion externally to halt the itching of eczema and psoriasis, and to heal burns, scalds, ulcers and to draw boils. Chickweed draws and absorbs poisons.

Recipes
Chickweed Cream

50 g (2 oz) chickweed
500 ml (18 fl oz) olive or sunflower oil

Infuse for two months. Add 50 g (2 oz) cocoa butter and 50 g (2 oz) yellow beeswax. Melt into the oil and cool the mixture slowly, beating constantly until it forms a smooth cream.

For external use only, as a cream.

Chickweed water for constipation
Add 3 x 15 ml (table) spoons of dried, or 2 handfuls of fresh, chickweed to 1.2 litres (2 pints) of water. Boil and reduce, until 600 ml (1 pint) remains.

Take a warm cupful every three hours until the bowels move.

Emotional uses
Being a water herb, chickweed is particularly appropriate for thin, dry and brittle people, who lack the flowing qualities of water, its compassion and receptivity. Such people tend to be self-contained, controlled and unspontaneous, and can do with the softening qualities chickweed possesses.

Drink a tea – 1 cup in the morning – for fourteen days and then stop. If you feel you need to continue, wait fourteen days and then repeat the process.

Chickweed is not helpful for, and should not be taken by, people who have very watery natures, who are plegmatic in temperament, where boundaries need to be strengthened rather than broken down.

Magical and ritual uses
Ritual for entering the wise age
The third aspect of the Goddess is the crone. After a woman's second saturn return (between the ages of 56 and 60) she enters the wise age and can be called a crone. Crones have an important function: they are keepers of the ancient wisdom, philosophers, soothsayers and grandmothers. Saturn is the teacher, the wise one, the mistress of time. She teaches us throughout maidenhood and motherhood, and by the time of the second return we begin to learn the darker secrets of life. She is Hecate, goddess of the wild

places, and Queen of the Night. Her colour is is purple. Celebrate this new stage of life with other crones. Deck the room with flowers of purple and white. Each woman brings a gift for the new crone. Something representing time: fossils, crystals, flowers or fruits of her colour. Toast the new crone: feast, sing, dance and celebrate.

CLEAVERS

Planetary ruler:
Moon

Qualities:
Hot and dry

Harvest time: *All summer*

Parts used: *Aerial*

Scientific name:
Galium aparine

Medicinal uses: *For the
lymphatic system*

Main constituents:
Silica, tannin, glycoside.

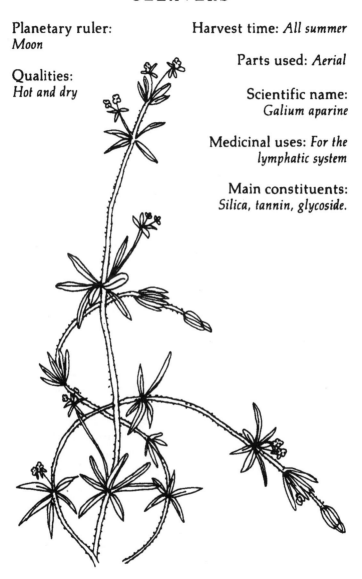

Myths and legends
Some of cleavers' names include: goosegrass, hedgeriff, hayriffe, robin-run-in-the-grass and everlasting friendship. The word 'hedgeriff' comes from old Anglo-saxon, meaning tax gatherer or robber.

The seeds are an excellent substitute for coffee, roasted over a fire.

Physical uses
This is a most important herb and anyone seriously involved in treating others with plants should have this remedy in her cupboard. It is the prime remedy for the lymphatic system which is concerned with the immune system of the body and fluid balance, and, as such, is applicable to many disease states, particularly chronic illnesses. Living in our polluted environments, eating junk food with chemical additives, which has been sprayed with pesticides, our immune systems are stretched to the limit, and when we are stressed or have low resistance we can become susceptible to viruses and other organisms. Cleavers works to clean out the lymphatic channels to strengthen and stimulate our immune systems so we can throw off infections easily. This is a remedy for long-lasting viral infections, for the debility felt after serious illness, antibiotic therapy or any kind of major chemotherapy, for instance, steroids or anti-depressants. It takes a few weeks to be effective but its use will build up stamina and strength and throw off the debilitating infection or effect of the drug previously taken. It can also be used for any disease of the lymphatic system, such as mumps or inflamed lymph glands. A lot of fluid is carried in lymphatic channels which, in certain individuals, for example, those suffering from excess cold, can build up into oedema (water retention) and cellulite (fluid retention in the thighs and buttocks as a result of faulty eating habits). Taking cleavers for at least a month will helpt to shift some of this fluid and reduce the waterlogging effect the latter has on the body.

Cleavers is also a diuretic in that it stimulates the

secretion of urine from the body. For this reason, it can be used to treat kidney stones, cystitis and urethritis. In men, it can be used to treat prostatitis. Besides mumps, this is a good all round remedy to use for childhood ailments such as chickenpox and measles, mixed with dandelion and meadowsweet. As it is a deep-acting cleanser, applied externally as a cream, cleavers can be used to treat skin conditions such as psoriasis (a scaly skin disease) and eczema and is sometimes of help in teenage acne. The silica in cleavers, a mineral found in grasses, is very healing, especially to mucous membranes (the tissues which line the mouth, gut, vagina and bladder) and is therefore useful where there is inflammation in those areas.

Recipes
A spring tonic

Take 5 g (⅛ oz) of cleavers, dandelion root and wormwood. Make a strong infusion of 15 g (½ oz) to 600 ml (1 pint) water.

Drink a wineglassful three times daily for a week.

Use at the beginning of spring to cleanse the body after winter's starchy diet and to prepare for the change of seasons which can sometimes herald sickness.

WARNING. It is not safe to take this tonic if you are pregnant.

Emotional uses
Cleavers is like a calm sea at twilight, the space between night and day, dark and light. It is that warm, safe place where nature seems to envelop, protect and subdue all the dramas of the daytime and yet not anticipate the mysteries of the night. It is a place of 'in-betweens' and emotionally represents the calm time before renewed activity, the hiatus, the pregnant pause before life begins again. It gives a feeling of peace, tranquility and stillness which envelopes the whole psyche, but it is not a sleepy peace, not a rest from exhaustion but simply the space between breaths, the inner

silence which we can fail to catch in the business of everyday life. Cleavers is for those about to begin a journey; a new phase; a change; a time to gather forces to allow recent experiences to assimilate and be made sense of, before moving on. Use for those who are in the process of change, who are moving on but need temporary respite. It is, however, not for those women who have no movement in their lives and who tend to get 'stuck' in one place.

Take cleavers tea for three nights before you set out on a journey. Ask for dreams which will help you on your travels.

Magical and ritual uses
Cleavers ritual

Cleavers is associated with the autumn equinox (21 September) and women gathering together to drum and dance – at a time when the seasons change and the inward-looking season of winter approaches. The women each dance their sacred dance of summer, dancing all the fire energy and inspiration it has given them, and with the rhythm of their bodies they take the energy inwards, storing it for the winter's coldness. The drums are messages to other women celebrating at that time and a rhythmic focus for the wild fire energy. It is a farewell to the light and a welcome to the dark side of nature. Women weave garlands of the last of the summer flowers and dance wearing them. After each woman has danced her dance, she throws the garland in the fire, saying:

> *The summer sun is dying.*
> *Winter draws in.*
> *Bring in the darkness of winter.*

4
HERBS OF JUPITER

Element: *Air*

Organ: *Liver*

Realm: *Judgement*

Humour: *Sanguine*

Function: *Digestion*

Qualities: *Warm and moist*

Herbs of Jupiter nourish and enrich the blood and the liver. They are often connected with the liver and its functions. With Jupiter there is a tendency to over-expansion, and the liver is the organ which has to deal with the excesses of food and drink. The liver also controls the condition of the blood and metabolism of the body (that is, fat, its production and storage) and the growth of tissues, whether healthy or diseased.

The herbs of Jupiter included in this book are dandelion, hyssop, lime, meadowsweet, melissa, red clover and sage.

DANDELION

Planetary ruler:
Jupiter

Qualities: *Cold and dry*

Harvest time: *Aerial parts from May until August; roots from November until March*

Parts used:
Flowers, leaves and root

Scientific name:
Taraxacum officinale

Medicinal uses:
For the liver, blood, kidneys and bladder

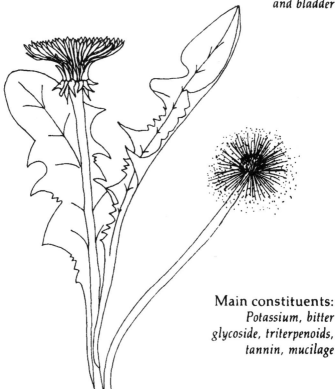

Main constituents:
Potassium, bitter glycoside, triterpenoids, tannin, mucilage

Myths and legends

The name *Taraxacum* comes from the Greek word *Taraxo*, meaning disorder or 'I have excited', and *akos*, pain, but also remedy. The common name 'dandelion' comes from the French *dent de lion* – lion's tooth – and refers to the shape of the leaves. It was also called *piss en lit* by the French – piss in the bed – on account of its diuretic qualities. Other names include: devil's milk pail and priest's crown.

Hecate was said to have entertained Theseus with dandelion, which is seen as a plant of Hecate. It is best to collect the root in November which is the month of Hecate.

Witches say that if you rub yourself all over with dandelion you will be welcome everywhere and that all your wishes will be granted.

American Indians used to smoke the leaf during shamanic rites.

Physical uses

Root

The root contains most of the bitter principles, so this is used mainly for liver conditions. As a bitter, dandelion should be taken before meals (say twenty minutes) to allow time for the herb to act. As a herb of Jupiter, dandelion root can be used for all diseases of the liver; it has been found to help build up liver tissues, so it may be used for hepatitis, cirrhosis, jaundice, gall stones and any kind of chronic liver congestion. As dandelion root helps the blood in the veins to circulate, it can be used with great success in cases of varicosed veins and haemorrhoids. (They are both part of the same circulatory system, so if the pressure is increased in the leg veins causing varicosed veins, it will also be increased in the rectum causing haemorrhoids.) It works as a blood cleanser and so can help in cases of arthritis, rheumatism and gout, as well as chronic skin conditions such as eczema and psoriasis, acting as an alternative working sympathetically with Jupiter to cleanse and regulate the composition of blood and, in the case of gout, removing excess uric acid from the blood stream. Dandelion root is a non-irritant remedy for constipation and works without causing spasms in the bowel, unlike senna and other purgatives. It affects all secretions and excretions in the body; it removes poisons from the system and can therefore be used for viruses and deep-seated chronic infections, glandular fever for example. It has healing qualities and has long been used as an effective treatment for duodenal and stomach ulcers. As it is a digestive stimulant, it can be used for indigestion, poor digestion, sometimes resulting in smelly feet, food poisoning, loss of appetite and other stomach ailments.

I have found dandelion root especially useful in cases of high and low blood sugar (hypo/hyperglycaemia), to help regulate the body's response to carbohydrates. Again, regulation of blood sugar can be seen to be a function of Jupiter.

Herb

This part contains more potassium and is less of a bitter and more of a kidney remedy. Dandelion herb is a powerful diuretic, useful to lower blood pressure and to rid the body of excess fluid. Dandelion herb will not deplete the body of potassium which happens with chemical diuretics which have synthetic potassium added if they are to be used for long-term therapy. Care must be taken not to give dandelion herb where the blood pressure is low as this will fall still further and may cause fainting and dizzyness.

Dandelion herb is a remedy for the kidneys and bladder; it is healing and soothing to the bladder, and is useful in cases of cystitis, urethritis and kidney stones. It also has an action on the lungs and can be used with other lung remedies in cases of chronic cough, asthma or bronchitis, to strengthen the lung tissues.

Recipes
Dandelion Beer

50 g (2 oz) dried dandelion herb
50 g (2 oz) dried nettle
25 g (1 oz) yellow dock

Boil in 3 litres (1 gallon) of water for fifteen minutes. Strain and add 1 kg (2 lb) of loaf sugar and 2 x 15 ml (table) spoons ground ginger. Allow to cool slightly and make up the liquid to 7.5 litres (2 gals). Add 15 g (½ oz) fresh yeast and stir in well. Ferment for twenty-four hours. Skim and bottle. It will be ready for use in two to three days.

Blood Cleanser
1 part dandelion root
1 part nettle leaves
2 parts elder shoots
2 parts primrose flowers and leaves

Steep 2 x 5 ml (tea) spoon of this mixture in ½ cup of boiling water.
Take twice daily.

To stimulate the metabolism
1 x 5 ml (1 tea)spoon each
alder buckthorn bark
liquorice root
dandelion root and leaves
pansy leaves

Soak 1 x 15 ml (table) spoon of this mixture in 2 pints of cold water for three hours. Bring to the boil and steep for fifteen mins.
Take 2 x 15 ml (table) spoons daily.

Emotional uses
The root, like all root plants, has a grounding and centring

action. Roots generally focus on the solar plexus and help to focus and ground emotions which are too scattered and too excitable. Dandelion strengthens the emotional body, gives the person a stronger sense of self, a clearer self-image and more power to resist the strong influences of others. From our solar plexus we create connections between ourselves and others, it is here that strong, often 'irrational', feelings we have about people are found. The instant dislike or great attraction we feel for others - psychologists call it projection because often these powerful feelings are our own repressed feelings which we cannot own for ourselves and hence have to 'project' on to others. As they come from the solar plexus, these emotions tend to be raw, intense and some-what undifferentiated; they are our basic demands and wants in our relationships. In love relationships, often the initial attraction is focused in the solar plexus - lust for example - but if the individual has the emotional maturity, it later moves up to the heart chakra where there is more impersonal, unconditional love. Relating from our solar plexus causes us to become entangled or tied to individuals which we might have outgrown emotionally. In her book *Motherwit* published in 1981, Diane Mariechild describes a useful meditation to check out the cords we have in our solar plexus and also a method whereby they can be safely removed. Dandelion root helps in this process by giving the person a strong sense of self; she can decide what relation-ships are really wanted and then let go of older, less healthy ties.

The root is also a bitter which describes how dandelion works on feelings of bitterness and hostility, to 'sweeten' the person up. Anger and resentment often get trapped in the liver and, if not allowed a channel of expression, turn to depression and self-hatred. Any herb which works on the liver will help, not only to ease the physical congestion therein, but also the emotional stagnation. Many, many times, after a woman has received dandelion or another bitter, she comes back after a fortnight, amazed and puzzled at how angry she has been feeling; generally the anger feels a good clean, purging kind, but it can be ferocious and explosive. For me, liberating angry feelings is vital on the road to self-discovery and liberation. As women, we need to reclaim and value our fury as the potent and creative force it is.

The root is useful to stimulate or excite those people who are the plodders in life, the dutiful, bound by conventions and fearful of change or innovation. Women who live their lives serving others: mothers of small children, carers of the sick and elderly, nurses, social workers. By providing a clearer sense of self and liberating their self-assertive tendencies, dandelion will empower such women to contact their needs and take some steps in having these needs met.

Take 5 drops of the dandelion root tincture for four to six weeks.

Magical and ritual uses
As a plant of Hecate, dandelion is used in the rituals of Samhain (Hallowe'en). Hecate is a goddess of the darkness, the crone, and her rituals are celebrated at the places where three roads meet. Offerings of fish, eggs and apples and pomegranates were made and rituals concerning divination or contact with the dead were performed. This is a time to remember the witches burned by the Christians, the night of the revengeful mother where scores can be settled. It is a time when women can deal with their feelings about patriarchal male violence and empower themselves.

HYSSOP

Planetary ruler: *Jupiter*

Quality: *Warming*

Harvest time: *July until August*

Parts used: *Aerial*

Scientific name: *Hyssopus officinalis*

Medicinal uses: *For the lungs and liver*

Main constituents: *Volatile oil, tannins, flavonoid glycosides, sulphur.*

Myths and legends

The Bible says 'purge me with Hyssop and I shall be clean, wash me and I shall be whiter than snow'. In those days hyssop was used as a purification herb; it was associated with the treatment of lepers and the purification of their houses. Hyssop was used in the consecration of Westminster Abbey. It was one of the strewing herbs in the Middle Ages. This meant that it was thrown on to the floor and then swept up with all the debris to clean and deodorise the house.

It is a plant much loved by bees and butterflies; beekeepers will always grow some hyssop near their hives.

The name 'hyssop' comes from the Greek *azob*, meaning holy herb because of its use in cleansing temples.

The oil of hyssop is used in the perfume industry as it has a fine scent. It is one of the ingredients of Chartreuse, a liqueur.

Physical uses

Hyssop is a cleansing lung remedy, useful for a wide variety of conditions such as coughs, colds, catarrh, sinus problems, nose and throat infections. It loosens mucous and reduces catarrh formation. It can be used as a gargle for a sore throat, swollen glands and tonsilitis. It acts on the digestive system and can be used to increase the appetite, reduce mucous congestion in the intestines and to treat flatulence. It has a slight laxative effect. It tones the mucous membrane lining of the gut and mouth and therefore relaxes any spasm or tension in these areas.

Hyssop can be used as a tonic for debility after an illness and to build up stamina. As it is a herb of Jupiter, it works on the blood as an alterative (blood cleanser).

Recipes
Queen Elizabeth's Cordial - Electuary[1] of Hyssop

Boil 600 ml (1 pint) of honey, skimming the surface frequently to remove scum. Add two handfuls of hyssop, well-bruised, and boil until the honey tastes of hyssop. Then strain and add 10 g (¼ oz) of crushed liquorice root, 10 g (¼ oz) aniseed, 5 g (⅛ oz) of both elecampagne and angelica and 7 ½ ml (1½ tspns) of both pepper and ginger. Boil for a short time and stir well. Remove from the heat and stir until cooled. Strain and bottle.

Dose: 1 x 5 ml (tea) spoon three to four times daily in warm water for seven to ten days.

For coughs, catarrh, shortness of breath and stomach ache.

For black and bloodshot eyes
Tie a small handful of hyssop in a muslin cloth. Dip into boiling water and place over eyes.

Oil of Hyssop
    600 ml (1 pint) cold pressed oil (eg. olive oil)
    25 g (1 oz) dried hyssop flowers

Let this mixture stand for one month.

Use to remove lice in humans and animals.

For earache, soak a cotton wool pad with the oil and plug the ear with it.

Emotional uses

I associate hyssop with the root chakra, with fear and being ungrounded. Use hyssop where the fear is extreme: for phobias, compulsions and obsessions. It is for those people who feel they are drowning in their feelings, who live their lives in darkness and cannot face the light of the midday sun; for those who need to develop more self-love and who cannot at present appreciate their own value. It is for those who do not know where their place in society is and need help to get a clearer sense of their direction and purpose in life. The base chakra is concerned with basic survival instincts, and if people are locked into their base chakra they are led by compulsions and addictions and are unable to enjoy any choice in their actions.

Make a tea of hyssop each morning before going out into the world. Take this for as long as you feel the need.

Magical and ritual uses

Hyssop water is used to scrub altars and sacred places and as a general purifying herb.

Meditation for dealing with a fear of life

Buy some hyssop seeds and germinate them. Water them and slowly allow them to come to life. Transplant them gently and grieve over those which cannot survive outside, for nature is ruthless. Go through the growth process with them, allowing them to come to full bloom. Value and admire these fruits of your labours and when they are in full flower, on the day and hour of Jupiter, pick them and dry them carefully in some sacred space you have. When they are dried, store them safely and use them for meditations or as an incense.

The meditation

Sit with the herb, either fresh or dried, and allow yourself to become at one with the plant, feeling your consciousness merging with it. Become aware of the chakra at the base of your spine. Focus your energy there. Feel the latent power and energy deep within you. Allow its heat and life force to radiate through your entire body. Stay with it for five to ten minutes. Come out and write about your experience. Do this meditation twice weekly for several months.

Ritual

Hyssop has associations with serpents and dragons and with the Kundalini energy at the base of the spine. Hyssop, whether drunk as tea, burnt as incense or thrown on ritual fires, can be used when this energy source needs to be tapped into.

Dragon day was celebrated twice yearly at the equinoxes, September and March. Not much is known of this rite except that in September the dragon was invoked, to carry fire energy through the winter, and was put to rest (or sent underground) in the spring as the sap was rising. The dragon is an ancient symbol of the fire goddess, representing dynamism, power, will and courage.

LIME FLOWERS

Planetary ruler: *Jupiter*

Scientific name:
Tilia europea

Medicinal uses:
*For nervous disorders
and the blood*

Main constituents:
*Volatile oil,
mucilage,
tannins,
saponins.*

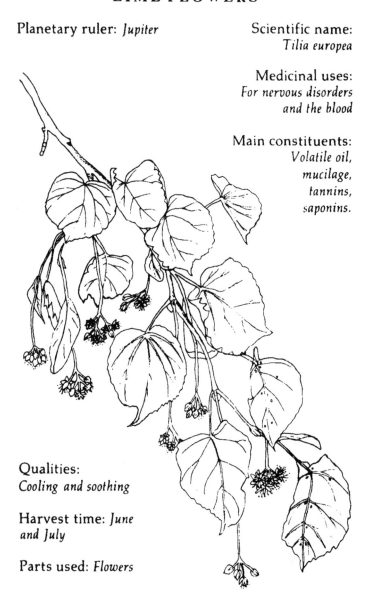

Qualities:
Cooling and soothing

Harvest time: *June
and July*

Parts used: *Flowers*

Myths and legends

The honey made from lime flowers (much loved by bees) is said to be one of the best in the world.

Pliny refers to the action of lime bark vinegar on skin blemishes. Hildegard of Bingen used a taliswomyn to ward off the plague – which was a ring with a green stone covering some lime flowers wrapped in a spider's web. Many old herbals claimed lime flowers were useful in the treatment of epilepsy.

Physical uses

WARNING. Lime flowers act as a powerful sedative which, when kept for over a year, have a narcotic effect. Therefore, strong doses of lime flowers should be treated with respect and women should not operate heavy machinery or drive a car after taking them. Even so, if you take lime flowers in doses greater than those suggested, they are not dangerous. You will just fall asleep.

Lime flowers are used in the treatment of hypertension. Many cases of hypertension are due to anxiety and stress and so a sedative will help to alleviate the increased pressure.

Lime flowers are used to reduce the effect of arteriosclerosis (hardening of the arteries) and therefore to reduce the severity of angina attacks. As a strong sedative, lime flowers can be used with great success in cases of persistent insomnia; a strong tea should be drunk half an hour before retiring. They can also be used for severe anxiety and for panic attacks as they relax the body and calm the heart, stopping palpitations. Lime flowers are useful for the treatment of addiction to tranquilisers and can be taken in conjunction with these drugs as their dosage is being reduced. Lime flowers are also used in cases of migraine, to stop an attack and promote sleep.

Lime flowers are sweat-inducing; use a pinch, together with a pinch of ginger at the beginning of a feverish cold to lower temperature and move the infection out of the body as soon as possible.

Recipe
A mixture to promote perspiration

> 15 g (½ oz) lime flowers
> 15 g (½ oz) elder flowers
> 15 g (½ oz) mullein flowers
> 15 g (½ oz) chamomile

Mix in equal parts. Steep 1 x 5 ml to 2 x 5 ml (tea) spoons in ⅔ cup boiling water.
Take hot.

Emotional uses

Lime flowers are related to the heart chakra. Drink them in a tea, whenever you feel the need, to calm and to centre and open that chakra. Lime flowers are especially good for those who give out more than they take in, who allow themselves to become depleted by their unselfishness and feel tired and jaded. They warm the frozen heart and allow for the rays of love to penetrate people who are cold and hardened to the world. They allow them to feel the love of others and to take that love inside themselves and thaw out from the inside. Lime flowers help the development of emotions from the solar plexus level of wants, demands and conditional love, to the heart level of love for humanity and a less attached form of loving, a more accepting kind. For people damaged as children by cruelty and coldness, lime flowers allow them to step out of that self-protective space and to include others.

Magical and ritual uses
For those who put the needs of others first

Make a daily ritual of brewing a pot of lime flower tea, as strong or as weak as you like. Do this at the end of the day because the flowers act as a strong sedative. Have a special pot and cup, and when drinking the tea remind yourself that your needs are important, and that self-nourishing is your priority. Remember that whatever is right for you and in line with your real needs is automatically right for those around you. Meditate on the warmth and honeyed taste of the herb and allow that heat and sweetness to fill your body.

MEADOWSWEET

Planetary ruler:
Jupiter

Qualities:
Warm and moist

Harvest time:
July and August

Parts used:
Flowers and leaves

Scientific name:
Filipendula ulmaria

Medical uses:
*For the digestive
system and rheumatism
in the bones
and muscles*

Main constituents:
*Salicylic acid, volatile
oil, tannin, mucilage,
flavonoids*

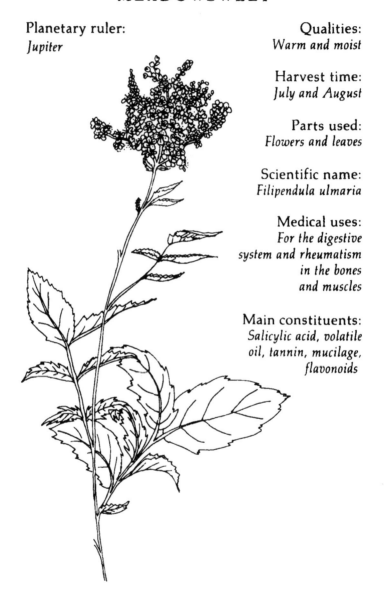

Myths and legends

Other names include dollof, queen of the meadow, bride-wort and lady of the meadow. Meadowsweet was one of the strewing herbs, used to cover the floors of houses to give them a pleasant, aromatic scent.

Meadowsweet, water mint and vervain were the three herbs held most sacred by the druids.

Witches used the plant in garlands in ritual and to protect their houses from evil influence. Somerset gypsies used the flower heads steeped in water, mixed with a little dew from the teasle plant, to clear the complexion.

Physical uses

Meadowsweet is *the* remedy for both stomach and duodenal ulcers as it decreases the secretion of the stomach acid and therefore the acidity in both the stomach and duodenum. It also increases the rate at which the lining of the stomach is renewed and so helps any ulcer to heal faster than usual. As a remedy of Jupiter, it increases the amount of bile produced by the liver and therefore works as a digestive stimulant, reducing any stagnation in the liver and helping the immune system to function more effectively. (In my experience, immunity is decreased when the liver is not functioning properly.)

Meadowsweet has an anti-inflammatory action and can therefore be used as a substitute for steroids.

WARNING. Steroids, like tranquillisers, can only be withdrawn under careful medical supervision. Sudden withdrawal may cause serious health problems.

Meadowsweet is used with great success in cases of rheumatoid arthritis, chronic peptic ulcers and any inflammatory condition, working to cleanse the blood of harmful acids. It affects the rate of which blood clots and so should be avoided where there are blood clotting diseases. Those who are on Warfarin or other anticoagulant remedies should also avoid ingesting meadowsweet.

WARNING. Insulin-dependent diabetics should NEVER attempt to substitute herbal remedies for insulin. Diabetics interested in long-term therapy must consult a qualified practitioner for advice.

The herb has an antiseptic effect on the urine and is a strong diuretic. It can therefore be used for kidney and bladder complaints. It acts as a painkiller and so is useful for arthritic pains and headaches. With any pain, however, the cause must first be established before measures are taken to reduce the symptoms.

Meadowsweet lowers fevers and is one of the best remedies for childhood infectious diseases such as chickenpox and mumps. If possible, use fresh or dried flowers in a tea to bring out a really good sweat. It has also been used with some success in cases of weight gain where there is a disorder of fat metabolism. This is sometimes found in diseases of Jupiter, which is the planet connected with cell nutrition and the laying down of fatty tissue within the body.

Recipes

Lotion for wounds
Make a strong tea of 30 g (1¼ oz) of meadowsweet to 600 ml (1 pint) boiling water and let stand for twenty minutes.

Apply after straining. It will keep in the fridge for three to four days.

Mixture for chickenpox, measles, mumps or any infectious fever
Mix together 15 g (½ oz) each of meadowsweet, dandelion root, marigold flowers and cleavers. Add 1.2 litres (2 pints) cold water. Bring to the boil and simmer for twenty minutes.

Take a wineglassful of this mixture three to four times daily.

If fresh or dried herbs are not available, use equal quantities of the tinctures and take 5 to 10 drops three to four times daily.

Emotional uses

Meadowsweet is a plant for those who have become too rigid, who need to learn how to relax and open out to life. The holding in may be due to fear or it may be because of anger, but in either case the person has constructed a suit of armour for protection from the outside world. Meadowsweet is a gentle opening out remedy; it warms and expands the psyche. Barriers and defences are usually constructed for a good reason and need to be let down carefully and gently. The herb diffuses and allows light into these prisons; it is uplifting as well as calming. It helps sensitive people to feel they can cope better with their lives; it strengthens and soothes.

Meadowsweet is especially good for young women who are frightened of their sexuality and feel overly shy and self-conscious. It can also help to straighten out feelings of fear and self-hatred following sexual trauma. I associate meadowsweet with the crown chakra, which connects us with the divine, our sense of purpose and with all life. Meadowsweet builds inner strength and helps to reconnect with faith and hope, for those who need to stand taller and more upright.

Put 15 g (½ oz) of dried flowers in a cotton bag and sleep with this sachet under your pillow.

Magical and ritual uses

Meadowsweet is associated with the festival of Lammas (1 August) a celebration of the Earth Mother in her form as Ceres Kore. The altar is dressed with bunches of flowers and fruits and the witches wear garlands of meadowsweet. Lammas is the celebration of the fruits of the earth and her abundance. Meadowsweet has a heady, narcotic perfume which helps the participants to leave their physical forms behind and contact the essence of the Great Mother and feel at one with her.

Meadowsweet tea can be drunk to heighten the effect of the celebration and to provide an atmosphere of merriment.

Meditation on the crown chakra

Pick a fresh bunch of meadowsweet, or buy some dried flowers or find a picture of the plant. Sit in a sacred spot and give yourself time to relax and deepen within yourself. Look long and carefully at the plant; if you have it hold it in your hands and allow yourself to make an image of the flowers in your mind's eye. Holding this image firmly in mind, feel the qualities of strength and diffusion that it has and allow yourself to embody those qualities. Feel strong but not rigid. Hold this quality for five to ten minutes and then write down what it was like for you. Repeat daily for fourteen days, noticing how the qualities of strength and flexibility are manifesting in your life and how you are developing the qualities of stillness and focus, and also how this connects you with the divine.

MELISSA (BALM)

Planetary ruler:
Jupiter

Quality:
Temperate

Harvest time:
June to
August

Parts used:
Flowers
and leaves

Scientific name:
Melissa officinalis

Medicinal use:
For the stomach,
heart and
nervous disorders

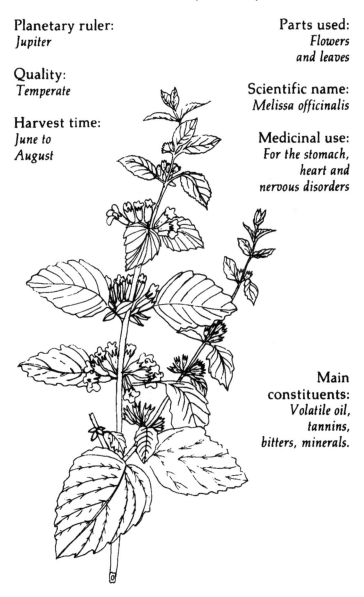

Main
constituents:
Volatile oil,
tannins,
bitters, minerals.

Myths and legends

Melissa, also known as balm, has a close association with bees and honey. Beekeepers used to rub the hives with melissa to keep the bees around the hive. Melissa means honey bee in Greek. In Latin America, melissa is called *tronjil para la pena*, that is, balm for your sorrows.

Melissa has the reputation for being an elixir of youth.

Paracelsus sold a secret melissa remedy to the Kings of Europe which he claimed was an elixir of life and that it prevented senility and impotence.

A tea of balm and marjoram was given to cows to recover from calving.

Melissa is said to increase fertility and has been used in love potions and as an aphrodisiac associated with rituals to Diana.

Balm is best picked on midsummer's day (21 June).

Physical uses

Melissa contains a volatile oil and as such is an excellent remedy for the digestive system, calming and soothing away the pains due to wind or tension, reducing diarrhoea due to anxiety and tension and gently opening the bowels in cases of constipation associated with depression or anxiety. The herb can be drunk as a warm tea for heartburn and indigestion; it helps the digestion of food, especially fatty foods, and so can be used after a heavy meal to prevent bloating and discomfort. It is an excellent remedy for those who are so tense they cannot find appetite for food; it helps to relax tension in their stomachs and allows the digestive juices to flow. It can be used in conjunction with other healing remedies (such as marigold and comfrey) in cases of stomach or duodenal ulcers to reduce the over-secretion of stomach acid and reduce spasm. The herb can also be used for mild tension headaches and for headaches due to gastric upset or biliousness.

Melissa improves the circulation and strengthens the heart and can be used together with other remedies in cases of high blood pressure or poor circulation. It can also be helpful in cases of vertigo and tinnitus, for palpitations and in pregnancy for headaches, dizzyness and morning sickness.

Melissa has been used as a relaxant remedy in asthma and stubborn coughs and for bronchial catarrh. It increases sweat production and therefore can be used to lower fevers and treat colds and flu or any low, recurrent fever.

Taken regularly, Melissa can regulate irregular periods, help ease the pains of menstruation and may be used as a slight uterine stimulant during labour to ease the pains of afterbirth. A decoction, poured into a bath and squatted in, will help to bring on a delayed period and ease cramps after childbirth. Melissa is also a valuable herb to take during the menopause: it helps with hot flushes, depression, anxiety and palpitations associated with the change of life. The herb regulates the circulation of blood around the body, especially to the peripheral areas, thus reducing the sudden changes of bloodflow which is the cause of flushes and sweats.

A bruised leaf, boiled in a little wine oil, applied to a boil will cause it to ripen and burst.

Recipes

Herb Pillow

Use 50 g (2 oz) each of hops, cowslip, migonette and melissa.

Stuff a small pillow with the well dried herbs. Renew yearly.

Queen Maria's Nourishing Broth

    1 chicken
    handful of parsley
    1 sprig of thyme
    3 springs of spearmint
    3 sprigs of melissa
    ½ onion
    1 clove
    salt
    enough water to cover
    Cook well and reduce to 600 ml (1 pint).

Take a wineglassful three times daily.

A refreshing drink for fever
2 sprigs of balm and a little wood sorrel. Peel a small lemon
thinly, slice and put in a stone jug. Cover with 1.75 litres (3
pints) of boiling water, sweeten and cover.
    Drink as required.

Syrup of Melissa (after Culpeper)
To every 450 g (1 lb) of melissa, add 1.75 litres (3 pints) of
boiling spring water. Pour on to the herb and stand covered
near the fire for twelve hours. Strain and repeat with the
same quantity of flowers. Then strain and to every pint of
liquid add 1 kg (2 lb) of fine sugar. Melt over the heat and
remove the scum. Bottled, it will keep about a year.
    Dose: 1 x 5 ml (tea)spoon in warm water three times
daily.

A purging electuary to purge melancholy (after Culpeper)
Powder the herb and pass through a fine sieve. To 25 g (1
oz) of powder, add 75 g (3 oz) of clarified honey. Mix well
and store in a pot.
    Dose to purge: 15 g to 25 g (½ to 1 oz) melissa. Dose as
cordial: 1g-5g ($\frac{1}{32}$ to $\frac{1}{8}$ oz) (½ dram-2 drams). Taken either
first thing in the morning fasting and having no food for an
hour afterwards, or before bedtime, three to four hours
after supper.
(To clarify honey, heat in saucepan gently until a scum
emerges; remove the scum and the honey is clarified.)

Emotional uses
Culpeper said Melissa 'causes the mind and heart to become
merry, and reviveth the heart'. It is an excellent remedy
for depression, sluggishness and negativity as Culpeper
notes when he says that melissa 'driveth away all trouble-
some cares and thoughts out of the mind, arising from
melancholy or black choler'. Taken as a tea, it will help to lift
gloom and despair and give some light into the person's life.

It will increase mental stamina and enable depressed women to concentrate again and allow their minds to absorb information, helping both focus and memory. It is soothing, warming, friendly, strong and yet delicate. It encloses and protects and allows for a sense of space to come into an individual's life again if she has been feeling trapped and hopeless. The herb is for those who need to be loved but are unable to receive, as well as for those who give out so much to others that their needs get put in second place, and for those who mother others and sometimes get drained and need to replenish their own stores. Melissa works on the heart chakra, opening out this centre and allowing for love to enter and for the possibility for unconditional love to exist. It helps habitual worriers, people who feel defeated by life. It is for those who feel aimless or are having a crisis of meaning in their lives. Melissa gives a person the ability to remain focused if many things are happening at once, and it is excellent in times of crisis to remain centred and yet open to whatever may happen.

There is also a strong sexual connotation with melissa, particularly for a woman who has experienced a sexual trauma of some kind such as rape, abortion, miscarriage, VD clinics or gynaecological procedures. It can help the woman to reconnect with a sense of being a woman unto herself and to rebuild her sense of inner integrity and wholeness.

Magical and ritual uses

A ritual after rape or sexual trauma

Invite women friends whom you love and trust. Each woman should bring a sweet-scented flower such as rose, melissa or honeysuckle. Fill your home with their scent and burn sandlewood incense and, if warm enough, open all the windows. Take a bath in which oil of sandlewood and melissa have been dropped. Visualise these healing, aura-cleansing oils washing away the memories of the pain, rage and darkness this experience has caused you. Light blue

A Woman's Book of Herbs

candles and send back all the poison, hatred and evil to its perpetrator. Return it to its source and know that good will triumph over evil, light over darkness. Chant the following:

May the evil of patriarchy be visited upon them;
may they know and suffer for what they do.
Blessed Be.

Take time to reaffirm your wholeness, beauty, purity and your ability to triumph over the cruelty of men. Have one or all of your friends sleep over with you that night and dream together a saner, safer, future.

RED CLOVER

Planetary ruler:
Jupiter

Harvest time: *May
to July*

Qualities:
Temperate and dry

Parts used: *Flowers*

Scientific name:
Trifolium pratense

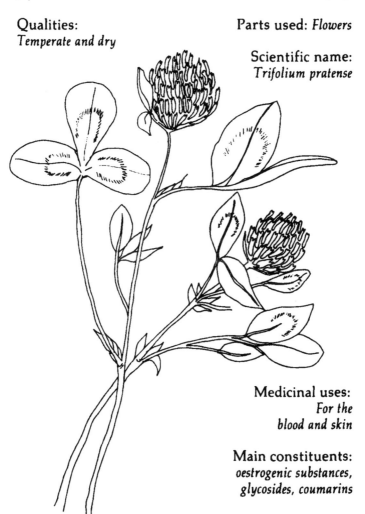

Medicinal uses:
*For the
blood and skin*

Main constituents:
*oestrogenic substances,
glycosides, coumarins*

Myths and legends

Each of the leaves of a normal three-leafed clover was said to represent one aspect of the Triple Goddess: one was the maiden – the young woman, one the mother – the fertility symbol and one the crone – old age and wisdom.

In other traditions, the first leaf of a five-leafed clover represents fame, the second wealth, the third faithful lovers, the fourth health and the fifth was said to represent bad luck.

Physical uses

Red clover is a deep-acting blood cleanser and as such is used in chronic, deep-seated conditions. Use in eczema, psoriasis (a skin disease characterised by peeling skin and inflammation), scabies and any other chronic skin complaint. It counteracts growth as in acting sympathetically it normalises or rebalances the growth of tissues, and is used for growths of the skin and the reproductive system.

Jupiter is the planet of expansion, or overgrowth of tissue. In malignancy, there is a rapid growth of cells and Jupiter can be seen as the planet largely related to the genesis of cancer, of growths, both benign and malignant, and worts and polyps. Treating the growths may include the use of the herbs of Jupiter such as red clover, which has a long tradition of being used externally to treat cancerous growths and ulcers and for relieving the pain of gout.

It is a relaxant for the nervous system and can be used for headaches due to stress and tension, and for spasms and nervous ticks. Drunk as a tea on a daily basis, it can be helpful for those who suffer from anxiety.

Red clover is a remedy for the female reproductive system and can be used in conjunction with other remedies for serious, debilitating conditions such as pelvic inflammatory disease (PID), endometriosis (a disease of the womb causing heavy bleeding) and very heavy periods. The tea can be used as a vaginal douche for thrush and other local infections and as a poultice or cream to soften milk ducts for nursing mothers and in cases of nipple eczema and mastitis.

Red clover can also be used for the lungs; it has a sedative action on lung tissue and is useful in debilitating coughs. The tea can be used as a gargle for sore throats. The tea stimualtes the actions of the liver and gall bladder and therefore can be used to increase the appetite and help relieve constipation.

The herb can also be used in a poultice for athlete's foot.

Recipe
Dr Coffin's Clover Salve
Fill a large saucepan with clover heads, cover with water and boil briskly for one hour. Strain and press and then refill the saucepan with new flower heads, adding the same water and repeating the process. Strain and simmer this liquid until it resembles thick tar, taking care not to burn it asthis will impair its virtues.

Apply the thick liquid to the affected area twice daily in cases of growths and swellings.

Emotional uses
Red clover is for those people who hold their emotions in and who hold things down, who have strong, negative emotions but are unable to release them. It is for depression, grief and sorrow. For worrying and over-thinking. It is my opinion that, when certain types of cancers develop, there is an attitude of mind in the sick person which seems to have some bearing on both the reason for the illness developing and the recovery from the illness. People who have many unresolved and unexpressed resentments, who hold hostility, jealousy or hatred deep within them and are unable and unwilling to let go of these feelings, seem to be the type of people who develop malignant cancers. It is almost as if the poisonous feelings cannot find expression in the outside world and, if they cannot be expressed and released, they turn within and poison the physical body. If this process is allowed to continue for many years, the body is eaten away with cancer. It has been found that those patients who are most likely to survive are those with a positive, healthy

attitude, who are outgoing and have a good social life, who have healthy relationships and who have something to live for, irrespective of the severity or mildness of the cancer. The Bristol Cancer Centre has done much excellent work in this respect, working with the physical body through diet, the emotional body through visualisation and counselling techniques and the mental body through positive thinking. It has some spectacular results using these methods, the 1990 research findings notwithstanding.

Drink a tea of clover flowers daily for as long as you feel the need.

Red clover works deeply and powerfully in the emotional body; it helps the person to be able to channel energy out, to express long-suppressed emotions and is fundamentally strengthening, providing a real boost to the life force. It helps to break through old patterns and gives vitality to pull through serious illness. It can be taken when it is felt there is no hope, that the darkest hour has come and all is lost; it can help to bring some light in a person's life. It is warming, soothing and restoring and helps to stabilise, increasing concentration and focus.

Magical and ritual uses

Clover was used in fertility rituals. At the New Moon (especially water or earth Moons)[2] when clover is in flower, collect several handfuls of clover in the morning before the dew has dried. Put them in a glass or crystal bowl, half filled with spring water, with a few drops of essential oil of sandlewood. Leave in the sun until midday, then strain and keep in a cool place. When the first evening star has risen, sit in front of your altar and light one white candle.

Invoke the goddess of fertility, the mother aspect of the Triple Goddess. Concentrating on the light of the candle, say the following invocation:

> *Cerridwen,*
> *Mother of all.*
> *Hear me now,*

calling to the spirit of my unborn child.
May it come to me
before the moon makes one circuit.
May it come to me,
blessed be.

Take the clover water and annoint your body, feeling the plant's healing strength and attractive qualities, and open your body to the spirit of the child. When the annointing is finished, collect up any remaining water and the candle and dispose of carefully, preferably in running water or at least far from your home.

Red clover was also used as a purifying herb to cleanse living and ritual spaces.

Steep 1 x 15 ml (table)spoon of red clover in vinegar for three days, strain and add to a bucket of good water (that is, sea water, spring water or filtered water). Wash your room, or, if carpeted, sprinkle liberally, to clear out bad influences (demons) and to be able to see witches. If you feel the space needs further purifying, put down a circle of sea salt on a plate or newspaper. In the middle of the circle, set a blue candle. Light this. Make sure it is secure, close the door and leave it to burn right down. Check the candle from time to time to make sure it is safe. When it has burned right down, carefully collect up the paper, salt and wick and take them to the nearest body of running water (stream, river or sea) and throw them in and walk away without looking back. If there is no such water nearby, dispose of the remains as far away from the house as possible.

SAGE

Planetary ruler: *Jupiter*

Qualities: *Hot and dry*

Harvest time: *July*

Parts used: *Flowers and leaves*

Scientific name: *Salvia officinalis*

Medicinal uses: *for ear, nose and throat, and the blood and for gynaecological purposes.*

Main constituents: *Volatile oil (30 per cent thujone), tannin, bitters, oestrogenic substances, resins.*

Myths and legends

Sage comes from the Latin *salvere*, meaning to be well, to save.

Ancient Latins had a saying about sage:

> *Contra vim mortis*
> *crescit salvia in hortis.*
> *Cur moriatur homo*
> *cui salvia crescit in hortis?*

Translated into English, this reads:

> *Against the power of death*
> *sage grows in the garden.*
> *Why would men die*
> *when sage grows in the garden?*

In the middle ages the herb was called sawge and was used for epilepsy, lethargy and the plague.

Traditionally, rue was planted amongst sage to keep toads away from this valuable plant. Toads were considered to be the Devil's familiar and hence a sign of evil.

In Buckinghamshire it was said the wife ruled the household if sage flourished in the garden. The prosperity of a person was shown by the thriving or withering of sage plants in their garden.

In parts of France the herb is said to be a plant which will mitigate grief, both mentally and bodily, and Pepys in his diary of February 1661 says that: 'between gosport and southampton we came across a little churchyard where it was customary to sow all the graves with sage.'

An old French saying goes:

> 'Sage helps the nerves and by its powerful might
> palsy is cured and fever put to flight.'

Billie Potts, in *Witches Heal, Lesbian Herbal Self Sufficiency* talks of sage as being a 'mother protectoress plant' and that it has deep associations with rites of passage.

Physical uses

As a herb of Jupiter, sage is good for the liver and therefore, as Culpeper says, 'it breeds good blood'. The herb is a deep-acting blood cleanser and a general tonic and tissue builder. It stops debilitating sweating, especially night sweats, if taken cold as a tea. It is a mood-elevating herb for nervous exhaustion and weakness, for headache due to tension, and for weakness in the sexual organs due to anxiety and worry.

Sage is an excellent remedy for all ailments which affect the ear, nose and throat. It can be used as an antiseptic gargle for the mouth and gums and as a strong astringent to help strengthen gum tissue. To prevent tooth loss due to weakened gums, rub the fresh leaves on the gums. It is also excellent for any mouth infection, pyorrhoea (gum infection), gingivitis (inflamed and bleeding gums) and mouth ulcers and is said to prevent dental carries if taken as a mouthwash on a regular basis. As a drying herb, sage can be used to great effect in cases of sinusitis and catarrh, to dry up excess secretions and free the airways from obstructions. It can also be used to dry up sweaty feet. As an antiseptic, it can be used in cases of tonsilitis, pharyngitis, laryngitis and sore throats. In this instance it it best taken as a gargle and swallowed afterwards. Culpeper, in *English Physician, enlarged,* suggests using a mixture of sage for the spitting of blood in consumption (p. 328). It can be used for pains in the head due to cold and cold rheumatic pains. The juice of sage taken in warm water is excellent for hoarseness and coughing.

Sage is an excellent remedy for the female reproductive system. It has the action of balancing the secretion of hormones and so is helpful both at puberty and during the menopause. Sage contains substances similar to the female hormone, oestrogen, which can be used to regulate the menstrual cycle if it is either too long or too short. Taken hot, it will bring on a delayed period, and for that reason must not be used in pregnancy. It is a remedy which stimulates fertility, especially where the cause is coldness in the womb or, as Culpeper says 'if women, who cannot conceive by reason of the moist slipperiness of their wombs [they] shall take a quantity of the juice of sage, with a little salt, for four days before they company with their husbands, it will help them not only to conceive, but also to retain the birth without miscarrying' (*English Physician Enlarged*, p. 328). If there has been a miscarriage, sage is a healing remedy to take and also helps to expel any material left behind in the womb from the pregnancy. It will dry up breast milk if taken as a tea, where the woman wants to wean or the child has been lost or in mastitis and breast engorgement; in such cases, take cool infusions for five to seven days. (If breast feeding, it is best to encourage frequent suckling with the baby correctly positioned at the breast – otherwise the milk might dry up.) For this reason, do not drink sage tea when pregnant as it interferes with milk production. Sage also helps to reduce heavy periods and slows down the rate at which blood is lost. It is especially useful in the menopause in the treatment of hot flushes, sensitivity to temperature changes and heavy bleeding. It can, however, be excessively drying and it is as well to put a Lunar or Venusian herb in the prescription to counteract excessive drying-out of the skin and mucus membranes (that is, the layer of cells on the internal surfaces of certain organs such as the mouth, anus and vagina).

As sage contains a volatile oil, it is also a remedy for the digestive system. It helps to reduce phlegm in the system and warms a cold stomach. (Phlegm, the fluid associated with the phlegmatic, tends to accumulate in the body, causing coughs and discharges.) Use for stomach weakness, poor digestion, to reduce vomiting and diarrhoea when these conditions become debilitating and excessive.

Sage is also a kidney remedy; it is a diuretic and increases the flow of urine. It is antispasmodic and restorative to urinary tissue and can be used to great effect in water retention, sluggish kidneys, gout, rheumatism and cystitis. It is a strong antiseptic and can be used both internally and externally for infection and wounds.

Sage is another herb that has been used to help regulate blood sugar levels and may be of use in both high and low blood sugar (hyper/hypo-glycaemia), but extreme care must be taken by those who are insulin-dependent if they use the herb so as not to upset the fine balance which has to be maintained.

Many herbs of Jupiter share this effect on the glucose levels of the bloodstream. It follows therefore that the action of Jupiter in increasing the size of the body fits in well with what we know about blood sugar, obesity and diabetes.

Recipes
Culpeper's Recipe for the Spitting of Blood

5 g ($\frac{1}{8}$ oz) (2 drams) spikenhard
5 g ($\frac{1}{8}$ oz) (2 drams) sage

15 g (½ oz) (8 drams) seeds of sage, toasted in a fire
20 g (¾ oz) (12 drams) pepper corns

Grind all these into a powder and add sufficient juice of sage to make them into pills and take a dram of them every morning, fasting, and also at night, drinking a little pure water after them.

Culpeper's Gargle

Take 5 g (⅛ oz) in equal parts of sage, rosemary, honeysuckle and plantain. Boil in 300 ml (½ pint) of wine to which some honey has been added.

Use to wash out the mouth, for sore throats and as a douche. You can add other warm herbs as required.

Mouthwash and Douche

20 ml (¾ fl oz) sage tincture
80 ml (2¾ fl oz) rosewater

Mix and use to gargle for sore throats, to gently brush gums with for soft gums and as a douche for discharge.

Use 1 x 15 ml (table)spoon of the mixture diluted in 300 ml (½ pint) of warm water, once daily.

Wash for breasts and nipples (after Dr Coffin)

Simmer fresh sage leaves in honey for thirty minutes, or until the honey turns dark. Allow to cool and apply to sore breasts and nipples.

Four Thieves Vinegar (used originally by grave robbers at the time of the great plagues of Europe)

Mix 1 x 5 ml (1 tea)spoon each of sage, rosemary, lavender, thyme and wormwood. Steep in 600 ml (1 pint) vinegar for one month.

Use to protect against infection; sprinkle in sick rooms and places which need disinfecting. Do not drink this mixture.

134

Emotional uses

Sage works on the throat chakra and is useful where there are blocks to expression. It can be used for those who have speech defects, who have something to say but cannot get the words out, for singers who need to loosen up blocks in their throats and for anyone who has something to say but cannot get the message over. Where there are blocks to creativity such as writer's block or for someone who has great fear of their own creative power, use sage as an incense or burn the essential oil.

Burn some dried sage – say 1 x 5 ml (tea)spoon – on charcoal each day, from Full Moon to New Moon.

Where emotions have been allowed to become stagnant, muddied, sedimented, instead of being expressed openly, often there is a need for catharsis – a need to express and re-experience the trapped emotions. Breathing and focusing on the feelings and/or the place in the body where the emotion is trapped can bring about a release – even though the feelings or emotions may be pre-verbal. It is sometimes easier to do this with someone else – a guide, therapist or friend who can facilitate this release. Unexpressed emotions such as crying, laughing and groaning can affect the physical body, especially the throat, the medium for vocal expression, which can become congested and may develop a disease.

Magical and ritual uses

Meditation to clear blocks to self-expression

Have a sage plant in front of you, sit before a sage bush or have a picture of the plant. Close your eyes and imagine the purple flower of the sage and see it vividly. Imagine this flower opening up to the light, bathing in the sunlight of a warm summer's morning. Feel the heat of the sun on the delicate purple petals; feel the flower gently expand to take in more of the light; feel it breathing in the goodness and health from the sunlight. Now focus on your vocal cords, they too resemble the flowers of sage. Imagine the warm light of summer sunshine relaxing, opening and softening these cords, imagine them expanding, opening out to the sunlight. Bathe them in the light and feel the healing power of sunlight revitalising and renewing their potency. Hold this image for five to ten minutes. Repeat daily for at least two weeks.

Rites of passage - death and her rituals

Death rituals are so important, and yet because of Western culture's desire to deny death and aging the process is associated with shame. We feel guilt and often a sense of failure, anger and frustration that the person is dying and has not been 'cured'. We have lost the vision which sees dying, living and birthing as part of a continuum, a cycle.

When it is clear that someone is about to die, remember that it is she who should be the centre of attention and not the grieving friends who can hold the departing soul back with their tears and lamentations. Light candles, bring fresh flowers into the room; wear white - traditionally white is the colour associated with death. Burn sweet smelling incenses and oils; myrrh, jasmine, frankincense and sage. Sit around the bed of the dying person and see her as a weary soul ready to separate from the physical body. See the white light of the soul rising from the top of the head and merging with the greater white light surrounding everyone. Sing, chant, hum as the soul separates from the body and the light moves upwards and away. Hold the focus of attention until the light has passed away. Open all the windows of the house and turn the lights on (if at night). Bring in flowers to surround the body and brew sage tea with honey. Serve some food and talk about the life of the departed. Stories, anecdotes, her best and worst qualities. Celebrate her freedom from her physical body and your friendship with her.

Notes

1. An electuary is a kind of syrup.
2. The earth signs are Taurus, Virgo, and Capricorn, while the water signs are Cancer, Scorpio and Pisces. See Lindsay River and Sally Gillespie, *The Knot of Time*, for a detailed explanation of the astrological signs.

5
HERBS OF MARS

Element: *Fire*

Organ: *Gall bladder*

Realm: *Imagination*

Humour: *Choleric*

Function: *Attraction*

Qualities: *Hot and dry*

The fiery planet Mars heats and dries all it comes into contact with. It resists poisons, cleanses the blood, moves obstructions, dries up the body fluids and stimulates the functions of the body.

The herbs of Mars included in this book are: bearberry, ginger, hawthorn, hops, nettle, vitex and wormwood.

BEARBERRY

Planetary ruler: *Mars*

Qualities: *Hot and dry*

Harvest time: *September and October*

Parts used: *Leaves*

Scientific name: *Arctostaphylos Uva-ursi*

Medicinal use: *For the kidneys*

Main constituents: *glycosides, tannin,
volatile oil, flavonoids.*

Myths and legends

Uva ursi means bear's grape in latin, and may have referred
to the fact that the fruit and leaves are so tough that only
bears can eat them.

The leaves have a high tannin content and were used to
tan leather in Scandinavian countries.

Being associated with courage and the warror self,
bearberry has connections with the ancient celtic goddess
the Morrigan, the Irish goddess of war. She was seen by
people as the ancient crone, gloating over the bloodshed on
the battlefields, drowning unsuspecting men under her
white waves and protecting her tribe, the Danu. She took
the form of a black raven and would fly over the battlefields
of the celts, appearing to those who were about to die. She
quarrelled with the arrogant Cu Chulainn warrior prince.
She offered him help in his battle but he scorned her,
contemptuous that any woman might be useful in warfare.
Her fury made the Morrigan resolved to repay him back his
insult to her. The following morning Cu Chulainn was
awoken with a war cry. He ran from his bed, naked, and
jumped in his chariot, only to discover as he fled down the
road that he did not know where the battle was. Confused,

he looked up and saw another wagon, drawn by a three-legged horse pulling the cart by a pole which ran striaght through its bright red body. Upon the seat sat a woman whose hair and garments were the colour of flame and her cloak the colour of blood. The warrior asked who they were but could not understand the answers they gave him as they spoke in riddles. He became self-conscious, realising he was naked and acting as a fool unable to understand his own language. The woman turned into a large black bird, cawing with laughter and flew off. When Cu Chulainn was next on the battlefield the Morrigan let loose fifty white heifers. She herself changed into one of them and led them through the battlefield until chaos ensued. Then she changed into a long black eel and twisted back Cu Chulainn's arms and legs, causing him to fall about; just as he was about to pull her off his body, she changed into a wolf and bit and clawed him until nightfall. Then she left him, hurt and bleeding. But she too was hurt, and knew the only way her wounds would be healed was if he blessed her thrice. She changed into an old crone and sat by the wayside waiting for him. As Cu Chulainn passed, the Morrigan offered him a cup of milk which he drank gladly, blessing her. She offered him two more cups and each time he blessed her. Having been blessed three times, she changed into a raven and flew off.

Physical uses

Bearberry is an excellent herb for acute kidney conditions; it renders the urine antiseptic and so fights any infection in that region by its action of resisting the infective organism, killing the poison in the way of Mars. Bearberry also heats up the bladder and kidney areas which may be easily affected by chills and dampness. It tones the urinary system, increases the circulation of blood to the kidneys, stimulates the action of the kidneys and helps to reduce accumulations of uric acid in the body. Use, therefore, for acute and chronic cystitis, gout, kidney stones, urethritis, nephritis (disease of the kidneys) and gravel (small stones like sand). It is said to work best where the urine is alkaline, that is, for those who are vegetarian, otherwise take bicarbonate of soda to make bearberry more effective – 1 x 2.5 ml (1/2 tea)spoon in water, if a heavy meat eater.

The herb can be used to treat arthritis with an associated kidney complaint.

It is a strong astringent and will help to check bleeding from the urinary system and the female reproductive system. Use for heavy periods, non-specific vaginal discharges, venereal disease and haemorrhoids. Bearberry dries out cold, damp conditions in the pelvic area.

WARNING. Because of its high tannin content, do not take bearberry for more than twenty-one days at a time. After this time, stop for twenty-one days, then, if necessary, repeat the dosage. By this time, it is best to consult a medical practitioner if the symptoms have not been alleviated. Don't drink black tea, also high in tannin, while taking bearberry. Avoid if pregnant and if suffering from nephritis.

Recipe
Mixture for Cystitis

> 25 g (1 oz) bearberry leaves
> 25 g (1 oz) thyme flowers
> 1.2 litres (2 pints) water

Mix the herbs together. Boil the water and add to the mixture. Cover and let stand for twenty minutes.

Drink over a period of forty-eight hours. After seven days, repeat until the symptoms disappear.

Emotional uses

I associate bearberry with the base chakra. Survival instincts, courage and great fear, comes from here. Bearberry encourages the development of the warrior within, and deals with victimhood. It helps to build a protective shield of armour, the ability to be self-protected and less fearful. It releases the primal energies of rage which may be trapped in the body as depression and allows for their expression. Conversely, it helps those who are locked in this raw, violent kind of energy to move up to a more loving and accepting place. People who suffer from addiction, alcoholics, drug or food addicts, operate from the base chakra. A woman, who may be mild and peaceable when sober, often turns into a violent, aggressive and unreasonable person when drunk. Alcoholism is the scourge of our time and increasingly a problem for women. Taking bearberry can help to cool violent passions and can lead the person to have a more healthy, balanced sense of her power and thus reduce the need for her to have power over others in order to feel safe and strong.

Burn 1 x 5 ml (1 tea)spoonful of the leaves whenever you feel the need, but not for more than three days running.

Courage is the positive side of the base chakra and courage is needed to be a woman-centred woman in this violent woman-hating world. The courage to stand up for what each of us believes is right, and not to follow the herd if we think it is wrong for us to do this. The courage to be our own women and to build new roads to travel down, to explore new ways of being powerful women.

If the base chakra is blocked, we feel a general fearfulness about life. Phobias are born here, as we cannot trust the world to be a safe place for us. We cannot trust the universe to provide what we need. Images of the warrior are often helpful in this respect, as they connect us to the sense of our personal power.

Magical and ritual uses
Use when undertaking occult work and to aid astral projection. Place leaves in an open bowl in the light.

Bearberry is used in incense to bring out the water element.

When the moon is waxing and is in a fire sign, the

following incense will help to balance the water element in the body when the body feels too watery (phlegmatic) and more fire is needed.

Mix 12 g (⅓ oz) each of bearberry, juniper, myrrh and dragon's blood, which is a red powder obtainable from herbal suppliers, in enough wine to make a thick paste. Spread out on tin foil to dry, leave for two weeks, turning often. Burn a pinch of the incense nightly.

The herb can be used as a taliswomyn to carry when there is excess fear.

Ritual for the warrior aspect

Warriors have never been needed as much as they are needed now in our troubled times. The warrior aspect of women is generally underdeveloped. There are battles to be fought; large and small, internal and external. Identifying with the warrior within engages our will to good, incites us to action, mobilises us.

A warrior is not the same as a soldier or mercenary who might kill for money. A warrior may be non violent and fight her battles differently. Greenpeace workers and Greenham women are warriors. Any campaign against injustice, cruelty and greed will involve the warrior within us.

Meet on a fire New Moon (in Aries, Leo or Sagittarius). Form a circle in the usual way and invoke the spirits of the four quarters, that is, the four cardinal points: north, south, east and west. Make sacred tobacco from bearberry, colts-foot, lemon grass and mint. Light in a pipe and pass around the group. As the pipe passes around, talk about the battles which need to be fought by each individual or in your community at large. Try to get a sense of the underlying struggle which the external events symbolise. Endeavour to go deep within the meaning of the struggle to discover its essence. Take time to explore the issue, allowing your abstract mind to see it from all aspects. Try to be creative in your analysis and explore possibilities. Devise a plan, a strategy for battling with this issue. Go through the stages of the will (after Roberto Assagioli, – *The Act of Will*)

1. *Goal-purpose-intention*
(What is to be done and why it needs to be done.)
2. *Deliberation*
(The pros and cons of this decision, whether or not it is realistically attainable.)
3. *Decision*
(The choosing of one course of action in preference to another.)
4. *Affirmation*
(Undertaking to carry out the decision and affirming your capability to do so.)
5. *Planning*
(Being specific; knowing what is to be done, when and how. Knowing what the first step is to be made.)

Share with the group your intention, affirm your decision and make explicit what the first step is for you.

Take a red candle, light it and out loud make your purpose known. Ask for the group's co-operation and support and dedicate your warrior aspect to the Goddess, blending your will with Her will.

Arrange to meet on the next full moon in fire, close the circle and bless and dismiss the spirits.

At the next meeting, repeat the ritual, this time discussing what has happened in the meantime. If the struggle has not yet been resolved, affirm your decision, look at any obstacles you may yourself have placed in your path and plan the next step.

GINGER ROOT

Planetary ruler: *Mars*

Qualities: *Hot and dry*

Harvest time: *October and November*

Parts used: *Root*

Scientific name: *Zingiber officinale*

Medicinal uses: *For the circulation and digestion*

Main constituents: *Volatile oil, resins*

Myths and legends

The creeping rhizomes (a type of root) of ginger were thought to resemble the convolutions of the digestive system and ginger was included in the Doctrine of Signatures[1] as being of use for the digestive system. Ginger has long been associated with dragons, their fiery breath and tempestuous temperament.

In Babylon the creation myth was about a dragon. In the beginning of the world when all was dark and formless, two beings appeared. The male was the spirit of fresh water and the void, and was called Aspu. The female, Tiamat, the spirit of salt water and chaos, was a dragon. She had the body of a phython, the horns of a bull, the teeth of a lion, the wings of a bat, the legs of a lizard, the jaws of a crocodile and the talons of a eagle. The gods were born of the union of Tiamat and Aspu. One of the gods killed his father Aspu, and in revenge Tiamat gave birth to monsters to prey on her offspring: demon lions, scorpion men, giant serpents and dragons. Chaos reigned. One of her sons, Marduk, was chosen to wage war on Tiamat. He caught her in his net and shot an arrow through her open jaws and split her heart. He divided her body in two parts and from them made the heavens and the earth.

Physical uses

Being very hot and dry, ginger warms the body which may have been chilled by an excess of phlegm (cold and wet) or melancholy (cold and dry). Use where the illness is caused by the cold: headcolds, catarrh, hayfever and for poor circulation where there is not enough heat in the blood to move the blood around – for chillblains, low blood pressure and dizzyness. Ginger is also for people who continually feel the cold. As Mars opposes Saturn, ginger can be used for the treatment of diseases of Saturn, that is, melancholy, aches in the bones and arthritis. Such treatment is called treatment by antipathy.

Ginger is a digestive remedy and helps ease the pains of flatulence and increases the flow of saliva.

It can be used as a first-aid remedy for menstrual cramps due to excess cold and damp and thereby opposes the action of Venus, working by antipathy.

WARNING. As ginger is an exceptionally hot herb, do not use where there is heat in the body: that is, with high blood pressure, stomach ulcers, inflammatory bowel diseases (colitis and Crohn's disease) as it will aggravate the condition.

Ginger reduces water retention in the body by increasing sweating.

The herb is diffusive, moving the heat from the head down to other parts of the body. It heats and mixes. It can be used where there is shock and collapse to get the circulation going, to increase fire in the body.

Recipes

Lemon Ginger Syrup

Bruise 100 g (4 oz) of ginger root and add to 1 litre (1¾ pints) of water and the thinly peeled rind of a lemon. Bring to the boil and simmer for three-quarters of an hour. Strain, and to every 600 ml (1 pint) of liquid add 450 g (1 lb) of sugar and the juice of a small lemon. Boil for ten minutes, then skim well. Cool and bottle.

Dose: 1 x 7.5 ml (dessert)spoonful in warm water, as required.

Emotional uses

Associated with the solar plexus chakra, ginger is concerned with feelings of action and reaction. Use for those who are cool, haughty and aloof, who defend their vulnerability with an air of superiority. For ice maidens to melt their wintry veneer. Also for those who are frozen in fear; some shock or trauma has shut down their warmth and spontaneity and caused a wall to be built around them. Gently and slowly, ginger warms the frozen feelings, relaxes tension and allows for an opening up to life, a beginning of trust. Drink a tea of ginger root whenever you feel you need warming up.

When feeling cut off or fearful, imagine the power and warmth of a dragon.

Magical and ritual uses

Initiation by fire

Put yourself in a relaxed, comfortable position. Take a ginger tea or syrup. Then take a few deep breaths, and breathe out any tension you are holding in your body.

Turn your attention inwards and imagine you are in a meadow on a warm summer's day. The sun is hot, a cool breeze is blowing, you are aware of birds singing in the trees, the drone of insects and the scent of flowers growing in this meadow. As you look around you, you become aware that there is a path in one corner of the meadow which leads down to the sea shore. Make the choice to follow that path down to the sea . . .

As you stand on the beach, watch the motion of the tides; hear the sound of the waves as they wash on to the land. At one end of the beach is a cave guarded by a wisewoman. She is the guardian of the fire of initiation which burns deep within the cave. Choose to walk toward the cave and make contact with the guardian . . . She leads you into the cave and you stand before the fire of initiation . . . Make the choice to merge with the fire, entering deep into its essence. Enter into the image and allow yourself to follow whatever comes up for you.

Slowly, in your own time, make your way back into the cave and then out on to the beach. Gradually allow yourself to come back into the room, and write down your experience.

HAWTHORN

Planetary ruler: *Mars*

Quality: *Temperate*

Harvest time: *Leaves and flowers – May; berries – October*

Parts used: *Flowers, leaves and berries*

Scientific name: *Crataegus oxyacantha*

Medicinal uses: *For the heart and circulation*

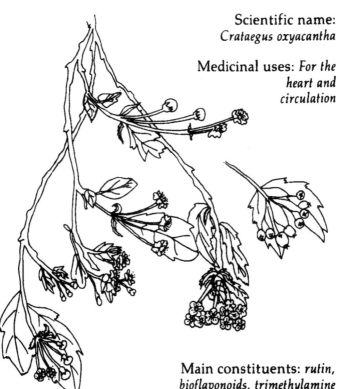

Main constituents: *rutin, bioflavonoids, trimethylamine (in the flowers only), tannins, procyanidins, ascorbic acid and saponins (in the berries only)*

Myths and legends
Country people believed the hawthorn blossom had the smell of the plague, and for that reason the tree was regarded as sacred.

A crown was said to be found hanging from a hawthorn bush which had come from the helmet of Richard III after the battle of Bosworth. It was for that reason that Henry VIII chose the bush as a heraldic device.

The berries were called pixie pears, cuckoos' beads, chucky cheese and ladies' meat.

The flowers were supposed to encourage fairies into the house, to bring good luck. It was considered unlucky to pick May blossom before the first week in May.

Hawthorn was one of the sacred trees of the Celts and was called Uath, that is, beauty, the tree of the sixth month.

The hawthorn blossom was called May blossom as it usually came out in or around May Eve, and was often used in the May Queen rituals.

The tree is also regarded as sacred because the Crown of Thorns worn by Jesus was thought to have been made from it.

Physical uses
The berries are used as the prime remedy for all heart conditions. They help the muscles of the heart to beat more effectively and move slowly and so the herb can help to regulate both high and low blood pressure. Hawthorn berries are used to slow a racing heart causing tachycardia (irregular beats), and to dilate the cornoary arteries in cases of angina to relieve the pain of that condition. Hawthorn berries have a healing effect on the arteries, improving their overall condition and rendering them less susceptible to arteriosclerosis (hardening of the walls of the arteries) and haemorrhage. In all these actions, hawthorn is working in sympathy with the choleric function of supporting the heart and the vital spirit which is the centre of all life.

Hawthorn, as a herb of Mars, makes the body more dynamic and rids the body of obstructions and blockages.

When there is water retention as a result of the failing heart, hawthorn berries can help to shift the fluid out of the body.

The leaves and flowering tops have a sedative action on the nervous system and also work on the heart and circulation in the same way as the berries.

Culpeper recommends hawthorn flowers for drawing out thorns and splinters; the tincture is best for this.

Recipe
To improve the circulation

10 g (¼ oz) dried hawthorn flowers
10 g (¼ oz) dried lime flowers
15 g (½ oz) dried melissa

Mix the herbs together. Take 1 x 5 ml (tea) spoonful of the mixture in a cup of boiling water. Steep the mixture for ten minutes. Strain and drink.

Dose: Take one cup daily for four weeks. Rest for one week and repeat the dose.

Emotional uses
Hawthorn works on the heart chakra and is especially useful where the person is full of anger and cannot express love, where there is a block to both receiving and giving love, or where love and caring are distorted into anger and aggression. It is for people with broken hearts, who are hardened and embittered after a failed love affair. It can be used where the person is very emotionally needy, sucking energy from other people and thereby pushing them away.

Sleep with a bag of some berries under your pillow.

Aggression and its constructive use
Aggression kills. It creates wars, distances and boundaries between women. It is hard to own and often gets projected on to others – for example, women who disagree with your point of view: white, Black, Jewish and Arab women.

Aggression traps us. Until we can accept our own violence, we will ever be beholden to it, frightened lest it shows itself behind our civilised facades. Owning up to accepting our own destructive aggressive impulses is the first step to being freed from its hold on us. As women, we have a convenient hook on which to hang all negative and aggressive emotions: that is, men. But women too have these feelings and, although they might be less often expressed in physical violence, they often erupt in emotional, psychological violence which, it might be argued, is even more damaging.

What then of aggression? How can we use this potent destructive energy creatively? Physical exertion in the form of dance or martial arts, running, screaming or shredding paper, pounding cushions with your fists or a tennis racket, all these things release build-ups of aggressive energy and allow for this energy to be transformed into something more constructive. Causes and political campaigns are another channel: marches, demos, letter-writing campaigns and sabbotage all release pent-up frustration and impotent rage. Spiritually, it means moving the fire energy from the personality level of the solar plexus to higher levels such as the heart or throat, so that the energy might be expressed in a less personal and emotionally charged way.

Using aggression in a more spiritual way is not the same as being nice. Righteous anger is a good and appropriate expression about bad conditions, and anger and outrage can exist without aggression. Ghandi was able to express his anger with the British without entering into battle with them. Likewise, Florence Nightingale and Mother Theresa had and have an absolute conviction of their rightness and peacefully overpowered those who tried to obstruct them.

This is the message of fire, energy, far vision, intuition and the right use of power.

Magical and ritual uses
Hawthorn ritual

Burn the dried berries as incense when you feel the need for more dynamism in your life. For courage to develop initiatives, to gain insight into problems, for clarity. As you burn the incense, focus your breathing on the solar plexus. Visualise energy moving from the solar plexus to the heart centre. From your heart you are able to see clearly problems in your life and what needs to be done to solve them. Thinking will never give you the answer to problems; you need to see the issues from a higher level, to find ways of resolving your difficulties. Seeing problems from the heart centre means they are seen with love, from a place of non judgement. This avoids blame or feeling guilty or ashamed about the situations we have got into. If performed a number of times, this meditation can shed light on the most intractable problems.

HOPS

Planetary ruler: *Mars*

Quality: *Temperate*

Harvest time: *September*

Parts used: *Flowers*

Scientific name: *Humulus lupulus*

Medicinal uses: *For nervous disorders and digestive complaints*

Main constituents: *bitters, volatile oil, tannin, resin, oestrogenic substances*

Myths and legends
Pliny spoke of the Romans eating the young shoots of the hop plant in the same way that we eat asparagus.

The leaves and flowers make a good brown die.

Hops are believed to engender melancholy. This is why it is unwise to use hops for counteracting depression.

The Jewish captives in Babylon drank a tea made of hops and in this way were able to stay clear of leprosy.

Hops were used as a remedy for venereal disease.

Physical uses
Hops open obstructions both of the liver and the spleen, by stimulating the secretion of bile and, as herbs of Mars, they cleanse the bloodstream of poisons. They have a laxative effect without being irritating. Hops are strong sedatives and are therefore useful for illnesses wnich are caused by stress and tension, for example, stomach and duodenal ulcers, and irritable bowel syndrome. Hops help to temper the heat of the liver and the stomach and are very useful for

headaches and sleeplessness owing to excess heat. Being a bitter remedy, hops help to stimulate the appetite and absorb food.

Hops have a beneficial action on the female reproductive system and can be used for painful periods. They increase the flow of breast milk in nursing mothers and calm infants who drink the milk of mothers taking hop flowers.

Hops increase the flow of urine and so help reduce water retention and they cleanse the kidneys of gravel and help to dislodge kidney stones.

Hop flowers can be used to treat fevers due to excess choler or blood (sanguine humour).

As painkillers, hops are useful as poultices used in earache, toothache, ringworm and any itchy skin condition, and they help boils and abscesses come to a head by drawing out the poison.

WARNING. It has been found that patients suffering from severe depression find their condition worsens when they take hops. If, therefore, you have bad depression or begin to feel depressed while taking hops as a remedy, stop immediately and consult a pratitioner.

Recipe
Herb pillow

Mix together in a mortar: 75 g (3 oz) lavender flowers, 75 g (3 oz) crushed rose buds and 75 g (3 oz) hop flowers. Add a pinch each of: lemon verbena, angelica and rosemary. Crush together with either 25 g (1 oz) powdered orris root or a drop of tincture of benzoin to fix the perfume. Fill a small cotton pillow with the mixture and cover with some bright fabric.

Herb pillows are good for invalids, babies and anyone who needs some help to get off to sleep. Renew each summer.

Emotional uses

There is a lot of sexual energy in this plant and its use can help women to become clearer about the true nature of their sexuality and the relationship between creativity and procreation, sexuality and love.

Sleep with a bag of hop flowers under your pillow.

Working on the womb chakra, hops can help heal emotional scars caused by the misuse of our sexuality. We may become involved in sexual activity when what we are really looking for is emotional contact, warmth, cuddling, physical closeness. Women who have been sexually abused, raped or have suffered cruelty at the hands of gynaecologists or obstetricians can help to heal these deep wounds by taking hops.

Take the tincture, as the tea is very bitter, over a period of several months, 10 drops daily, and make time to note any dreams, images, memories and feelings which arise.

Magical and ritual uses

Hops ritual

In modern astrology, Mars represents sexuality whereas Venus is seen as the planet of love. The ancients knew otherwise and saw Venus as both sex and love and Mars governing warfare. Strongly Venusian types were prone to venery (that is, hunting – the chase) and likely to catch venereal disease because of their indiscriminate unbounded sexuality, whereas Martian individuals were seen to have the self-discipline of soldiers to choose the appropriate time to fight or make love. 'Make love not war' was a battlecry of the 1960s. But indiscriminate sexual activity has lead, via the scares of herpes and penicillin-resistant gonorrhoea, to cervical cancer and AIDS and a multi-million pound porn industry which corrupts and exploits children and adults alike. Sexuality is a powerful but now potentially deadly impulse, a potent form of self-expression, a means of control and it may express the finest feelings in the human heart. From the mountain tops to the gutters and back again, many are slaves to its vices, its honeyed promise . . . and baffled by its disappointing ordinariness.

Sex and magic have a long history. It is said Atlantis fell because the priestesses abused their knowledge of sex and magic and the sacred became profane and all was lost. The vestal virgins took it as their sacred duty to lie with a stranger once a year in the service of the Goddess. They were virgins in the ancient meaning of the word - that is, women unto themselves who bore no allegiance or exacted no support from any man. This of course precluded any knowledge of the father so the patriarchal culture soon debased the practice, calling these women prostitutes as if such favours were for the buying and selling. Now, women have more sexual freedom than every before . . . and yet sexuality is a minefield. Both lesbian and heterosexual behaviour leaves much to be desired and one is forced to ask 'whither love'? But celibacy, too, is said to harden the heart and quell the vital spirit. Old philosophers said love was a form of madness and that sexual passion clouded our reason and made brutes of us.

Meditation on sexuality

Find a quiet spot where you will be undisturbed for half an hour. Lie down and take a few deep breaths to relax your body and calm your mind. Taking your awareness deep inside you, focus on your womb. See in front of you a door marked sexuality. Look at the condition of the door. Does it look well cared for or neglected? If you are willing, open the door and make your way down the steps on the other side. You will meet a wise person on the other side who will guide you. Follow him or her, and, as you are lead, ask any questions you need to ask. Take some time to really explore this world. When you feel ready, pass through the door again and slowly return to consciousness. Write down what happened to you.

STINGING NETTLES[2]

Planetary ruler: *Mars*

Qualities: *Hot and dry*

Harvest time:
May to September

Parts used: *Aerial*

Scientific name: *Urtica dioica*

Medicinal uses:*For the
blood and the skin*

Main constituents:
*tannin, iron, histamin,
gluconins, vitamins
A, B, C and K.*

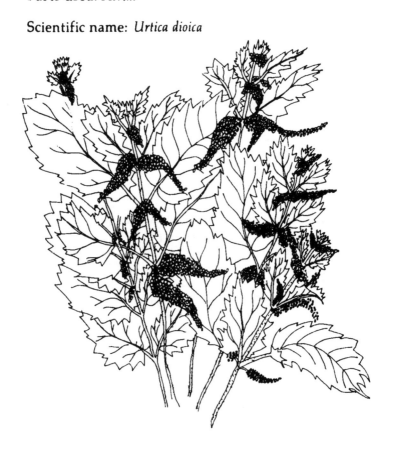

Myths and legends

The name *Urtica* comes from the Latin *uro*, I burn. The Anglo-Saxon name for nettle was *noedl*, meaning needle.

Long ago, nettle was said to be an antidote to hemlock, mushrooms and mercury, as well as an antidote to henbane, serpents and scorpions.

In France it was believed that if nettle and yarrow were held in the hand together they would quell fear.

Nettle plants were encouraged to grow next to roses to keep green and black fly away, and next to plants high in essential oils (the aromatic herbs) to increase their essential oil content. The herb can be hung in the house to keep flies away.

An old rhyme goes:

> *'Nettle in, dock out*
> *dock rub nettle out!'*

referring to the effect of rubbing dock leaves on a nettle sting to stop the pain.

It is believed that Roman soldiers who suffered badly from the cold wet British weather, used to rub themselves with nettles to keep their joints warm and mobile.

Nettle can be used to weave cloth and was used for that purpose as late as the seventeenth century in Scotland. The fibre from nettle was also used as twine for fishing nets.

Physical uses

Nettle, being hot and dry, rids the body of phlegm and was traditionally taken as a spring cleanser to clear the body of phlegm which accumulated during the winter rains. Culpeper suggests that as it is made into an electuary, nettle opens the lungs and allows trapped phlegm to escape. So it should be used in asthma, wheezing, mucousy bronchitis and catarrh. Drunk as a tea or gargled with, nettle helps to relieve inflammations of the throat, such as tonsillitis and laryngitis. The fresh juice, taken three days' running, stops bleeding gums. Being hot and dry, nettle is used to treat skin irritations and may be used in eczema, urticaria (stinging), heat rash, boils, acne and any hot, dry itchy skin diseases.

The tannin contained in the herb makes nettle a strong astringent and therefore excellent for haemorrhages anywhere in the body. It is used for heavy periods, bleeding after childbirth, nose bleeds and as a poultice for wounds.

Nettle is an excellent herb to take in late pregnancy; its high iron content will regulate haemoglobin levels and prevent anaemia and it also stimulates the production of breast milk. Use at any time when there has been loss of blood and the person is anaemic. Its Martian aspect increases the iron content of the blood.

Nettle is a powerful diuretic and is used in Europe to clear the body of uric acid which is found in high quantities in the bloodstream with arthritis and rheumatism. It is therefore a powerful remedy for gout, arthritis and rheumatism.

The powdered seeds have been used with some success in goitre (swelling of the thyroid gland) and weight (obesity) problems.

Recipes
Electuary of Nettle

Beat some dried nettle leaves into a fine powder and pass through a hair sieve to remove any large particles. To 25 g (1 oz) of powder, add 75 g (3 oz) of clarified honey and mix well in a mortar. Store in an earthenware pot.

Dose: 15 g to 25 g (½ to 1 oz) to purge the body of phlegm.

Nettle Beer

Mix together
A bucketful of nettle leaves
3-4 handfuls of dandelion tops
3-4 handfuls of cleavers
25 g (1 oz) bruised ginger

Boil together with 7.5 (2 gallons) of water for fifteen minutes and then strain. Add brown sugar and, while still warm, float a piece of toast on the liquid with yeast spread on it and 1 x 5 ml (1 tea)spoon sugar. Keep warm for six to seven hours. Remove the scum and add 1 x 5 ml (1 tea)spoonful of cream of tartar. Bottle.

Take for the pain of gout and rheumatism.

Nettle Pop
Boil the fresh young tops in a gallon of water with the juice of 2 lemons, 1 x 5 ml (1 tea)spoon of crushed ginger and 450 g (1 lb) of brown sugar. Cool and float a piece of toast with yeast spread on it to ferment. Strain, skim and bottle.

Gypsy remedy for aching joints
Take bunches of nettle and beat on the sore joint until great heat has been produced. Then apply cotton cloths previously soaked in vinegar. After several hours repeat.

Nettle Pudding

3.5 litres (1 gallon) nettle tops
2 large leeks
2 heads broccoli
100 g (4 oz) rice

Chop the vegetables and mix with the nettles. Spread a layer of vegetables on a large piece of muslin, then a layer of rice, and repeat until all the ingredients have been used up. Tie tightly and boil in salted water, long enough to cook the rice and vegetables (about twenty minutes).

Serve with melted butter. For four to six people.

For lusterless hair

2 handfuls of nettle tops simmered in 1.2 litres (2 pints) of vinegar and water for two hours. Strain and bottle. Saturate the scalp with the mixture every night.

Emotional uses

Nettle builds and empowers the fire element in a person, and helps to break up excessive watery or waterlogged emotions to allow the person to contact her rage and anger and cut through self-pity and victimhood. It is for evoking the will in women and contacting the warrior within. Nettle will warm a frozen heart and allow for the passion and intensity of fire to blaze forth. It gives a tensile strength to the emotions, rendering them less fragile or overpowering, and allows the woman to contact her own inner resources and feel her own power and resilience.

Drink a cup of nettle tea every day in the morning. Continue for as along as you feel the need.

Magical and ritual uses

If you have a way with herbs, like solitude, the silence of a moonlit sky, and can affect events by visualising them, then there is no doubt you are already a witch, whether or not you know this. To me witches are warriors. Witchcraft has always been the tool of the opressed. Via secret, occult means, witches have been able to protect themselves; to heal, to divine the future and to have access to power. For this reason, workers in magic have always, and still are, persecuted, particularly by the established church, by governments and whoever represents the status quo. It states clearly in the Bible 'The crime of witchcraft is the crime of rebellion' (book of Samuel).

The practice of witchcraft is a revolutionary act with its intent to remove the patriarchal state and replace it with an equal and just rule of law. To be a witch is to make a political statement. It is more than a religious affinity to a female diety; it represents a challenge to male-identified logical linear thinking. It is a subversive act, asserting the existence of another more complete, more wholesome, reality. Witchcraft makes us strong, independent, creative, thoughtful women. It connects us with life, with the earth and its cycles, and with all other witches, both esoterically

and exoterically (that is, hidden and open), wherever they might be working. To become a witch:
say:

> *I am a witch*
> *I am a witch*
> *I am a witch*

and you will be. Blessed be.

Nettle is a plant for the witch's tool bag. Drink it, grow it, burn it as incense. May patriarchy fall!

VITEX

Planetary ruler: *Mars*

Qualities: *Hot and dry*

Harvest time: *October*

Parts used: *Berries*

Scientific name: *Vitex agnus castus*

Medicinal uses: *For gynaecological
conditions*

Main constituents: *Hormonal-like
substances*

Myths and legends
Other names for vitex include chaste berry and monk's
pepper, which refer to its effects on the libido as it slightly
lowers the sexual drive.

Athenian matrons in the sacred rites of Ceres used to
string their couches with vitex leaves. Ceres was seen as
Mother Earth, as the earth-ruling part of the trinity with
Juno, the queen of heaven, and Persephone, queen of the
underworld. She was called Ceres Legifera, the make of
laws, and she was considered to be the founder of the
Roman legal system. She ruled Rome some time during the
four centuries before 200 BC, the written documents of
which were later destroyed by patriarchal vandals. Farmers
saw Ceres as the source of all food and kept her rites lest the
crops should fail. Her festival, Cerealia, was celebrated as
late as the nineteenth century in Britain; in the middle of
June farmers went round their corn with burning torches
in her memory. J.G. Frazer in the *Golden Bough* (p. 527) tells
of a custom in France where the last sheaf of corn becomes
the Corn Mother and is made into a figure of a woman. She
was dressed in clothes belonging to the farmer and given a
crown and a blue or white scarf. At the dance in the

evening, the fastest reaper danced around the figure with his girl. A pyre was made; all the women wearing wreathes stripped the Corn Mother and pulled her to pieces and she was thrown on the pyre along with their wreaths. The woman who finished reaping first set fire to the pyre and all prayed to Ceres to give them a good harvest next year.

Physical uses

Vitex is believed to work on the pituitary gland of the body and helps to regulate the hormonal secretions of the female reproductive system. It is the remedy of choice for the treatment of PMA (pre-menstrual awareness), for irregular periods, heavy periods and menstrual cramps. I have used it several times to prevent miscarriage in an otherwise normal pregnancy and also to promote ovulation. Where there is infertility, vitex will help to stimulate conception. Vitex also helps to clear premenstrual migranes and it regulates the menstrual cycle in women who have taken the pill as well as those who have chronic thrush – especially if this is a side effect of the pill. It can clear up acne which begins at puberty, especially if it seems to be related to their menstrual cycle. With migraine which occurs at ovulation or premenstrual migraine, vitex is the herb of choice. It will help to bring on an irregular period or will start periods again if for any reason they have stopped. Vitex can also be taken by women at the menopause if common symptoms of the menopause (hot flushes, night sweats and vaginal dryness) are partricularly severe. it works by antipathy to the Moon and Venus, opposing their excess wateriness and coldness, reducing secretions such as blood and heating the womb and ovaries sufficiently for life to exist.

In my experience, a precise mixture of Mars, Venus and the Moon is needed for conception to occur. Too little of one of those planets or too much of another will prevent conception or will cause miscarriage. If there is too much Venus or Moon, the womb becomes too slippery and the seed cannot embed itself in the womb lining. Conversely, if the womb is too hot and dry, the seed dies for lack of nourishment. Analagies to gardening are indeed highly appropriate when considering conception and pregnancy, and to a large extent the same rules apply. A well-nourished soil with sufficient vitamins and minerals provided, with enough sunlight, rain and drainage, will enable the seed to germinate. So it is with human fertilised seeds taking root in the womb.

Take vitex in tincture form. It has been found that it works best if taken first thing in the morning when the pituitary gland is most active. Take 15 drops before breakfast daily. It must be taken for at least one menstrual cycle for any results to be seen and generally needs to be taken for at least six months and then gradually withdrawn by lowering the dose bit by bit.

After a miscarriage, take 15 drops every half an hour and stay in bed. When the bleeding subsides, take 15 drops six times daily for another two weeks. Miscarriage is most likely in the first twelve weeks of pregnancy, especially at the time when your period would have been due. If you are having amniocentesis and are worried about miscarriage, take 15 drops of vitex first thing in the morning, for one week beforehand and one week afterwards.

Emotional uses

Just as Ceres represents life, so death is an ever present theme with adult women. Death in childbirth, the death of babies and children, death by rape and murder, death of part of the mother herself when the first child is born. The beginning of womanhood, the end of maidenhood, the experience of mothering – whether your child lives or dies, she or he is always with you.

The words of an Abyssinian woman sum up the relationship between a woman and her body:

The woman is from the day of her first love another. That continues so all through life. The man spends a night by the woman and goes away. His life and body are always the same. The woman conceives. As a mother she is another person than the woman without child. She carries the fruit of the night for nine months in her body. Something grows. Something grows into her life that never again departs from it. She is a mother. She is and remains a mother even though her child die, though all her children die. For at one time she carried the child under her heart. And it does not go out of her heart ever again. Not even when it is dead. All this the man does not know; he knows nothing. He does not know the difference before love and after love, before motherhood and after motherhood. He can know nothing. Only a woman can know that and speak of that. That is why we won't be told what to do by our husbands.[3]

Take vitex daily (15 drops in the morning) when you feel damaged or distressed about your womb. After miscarriage abortion, surgery, difficult childbirth or the death of a child.

If you have experienced the death of a child, make yourself a bath with the vitex seeds. Put 1 x 15 ml (table)spoonful of the seeds in a cotton or muslin bag and tie under the hot water tap. Allow the hot water to run through the bag, making a kind of tea. Lie in the bath for ten to fifteen minutes, preferably in candlelight, allowing the healing seeds to draw out some of the grief your body is holding in. Repeat nightly, whenever you feel the need.

Magical and ritual uses

The Festival of Lammas on 1 August was dedicated to Ceres. The altar is dressed with the fruits of the earth: flowers, grapes, corn and other grains. The candles are green for material well-being. Branches of any grain are used for crowns. A prayer of thanks is made to the earth mother for the fruits of her body, and a wish that all her followers might be kept fed and sheltered in the coming year. A libation is made and special food is laid out for her; the celebrants feast and entertain the goddess with song and dance and poetry and the fruits of women spirit.

WORMWOOD

Planetary ruler: *Mars*

Qualities: *Hot and dry*

Harvest time:
August

Parts used:
Whole plant

Scientific name:
Artemisia absinthium

Medicinal use:
*For the liver
and the blood*

Main constituents:
*Volatile oil (thujone),
a bitter (absinthin),
silica,
vitamins B and C.*

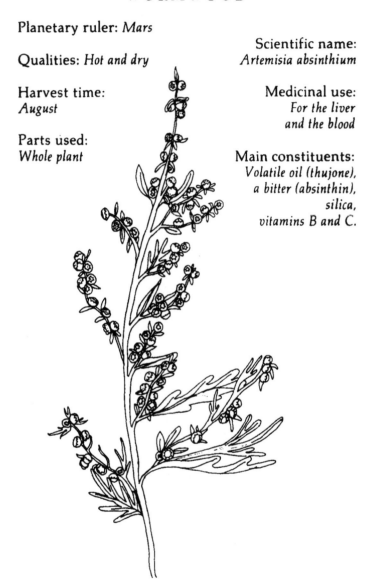

Myths and legends

In Russia it was believed that the bitter taste of wormwood was due to the plant's absorption of all human suffering from the soil.

In the eighteenth century in England a toast to happiness included wormwood in the mixture.

Pliny said that if travellers kept some wormwood on their bodies, especially in the shoes, they would not suffer from fatigue as it stimulated the circulation.

Mexicans celebrated the great festival of the Goddess of Salt by a ceremonial dance of women wearing a garland of wormwood.

Wormwood was an ingredient of a love charm.

In the herbal of Apuleius Platonicus (around 1000AD) it is said that wormwood was discovered by Diana who gave it to the healer Chiron.

Physical uses

Wormwood is a powerful bitter and as such is used for all liver complaints: jaundice, hepatitis, gall stone and cirrhosis. It is also used in the treatment of alcohol and drug abuse. As a herb of Mars, it resists poisons and builds up the body's immune system and so is useful in the treatment of viruses, chronic infections and infestation with parasites. Wormwood kills worms and can be used for that purpose in both animals and humans. It clears blockages and obstructions as a result of phlegm (that is, catarrh, vaginal discharges – leucorrhoea – and sinus problems) and cleans the blood. It opens the pores of the body and promotes perspiration.

WARNING Wormwood is dangerous if used over long periods of time, so never use for more than three weeks consecutively. Do not exceed the recommended dose.

Culpeper on wormwood

'Wormwood is a herb of Mars . . . It is hot and dry in the first degree, viz. Just as hot as your blood, and no hotter. It remedies the evils Choler can inflict on the Body of Man by

Sympathy. It helps the evils of Venus and the wanton girl produce by Antipathy . . . it cleanseth the body of choler . . .'
(From *The English Physician Enlarged*)

Recipes
Trotula reports that Galen, who was born in AD 131 in Asia Minor, practised as a surgeon in Rome and wrote eighty-three books on medicine, suggested steeping wormwood in wine and taking it warm for retained and delayed periods.

Trotula's recipe for delayed periods

Mix together:
10 g (¼ oz) wormwood
10 g (¼ oz) sage
10 g (¼ oz) pennyroyal
Honey (enough to mix into a paste)
Soak a piece of wool or cloth in the mixture and apply to the stomach.

Trotula's recipe for menstrual pain
Mix together 2.5 g (1/16 oz) (1 dram) each of betony, pennyroyal and wormwood. Add to a mixture of wine and water. Simmer and reduce liquid to half the volume and drink hot.

To speed up labour (after Trotula)

Mix together:
10 g (¼ oz) rue
10 g (¼ oz) mugwort
10 g (¼ oz) wormwood
600 ml (1 pint) oil
1 x 5 ml (1 teasp) sugar
Simmer for thirty minutes, making sure the oil does not overheat. Strain and rub over the womb area.
It will stimulate muscle contractions and get things going.

A poultice for mastitis (after Trotula)
Mix together the following in powdered form:
10 g (¼ oz) mallow
10 g (¼ oz) mistletoe
10 g (¼ oz) wormwood
10 g (¼ oz) mugwort

Add grease. Rub over the nipple.

Emotional uses
Wormwood gives courage, daring, fearlessness and ruth-lessness. It engenders a zest for life for those who are depressed, lethargic and slow. For people who are angry but are unable to express this anger, it allows them to open out. It has the effect of shattering form and then putting it back together.

WARNING. Wormwood is a strong herb and should not be given to uncentred people, or to those suffering from grief or shock.
Give to those who are dying, to enable them to let go and die in peace.
Make a taliswomyn of wormwood and carry it with you.

Magical and ritual uses
Wormwood is a herb of the magician/shaman and has particular affinity for the desert. It is used in initiation rites, for tests of courage and daring, and for preparing for journeys into the unknown.
Shamans are said to be chosen and not elected as is the case with witches. Often they are born with an extra bone, finger or toe. They are sometimes 'summoned' during a serious or life threatening illness, often occuring in child-hood. The shaman returns from the illness transformed. Sometimes there is no memory of the previous life, the name, family or any details. Recovery can be dependent on the person undertaking to do the shamanic training and to subsequently heal this illness. During the initiation the

shaman is disembodied and her body scattered to the four winds. She is then reassembled but is forever changed. The shaman confronts her own fear (called by some The Dweller on the Threshold), battles with it and emerges triumphant. Shamans are healers who take on the sickness of the individual or group, transform and interpret it. They often have a catalytic effect on people and situations and generally travel alone. They use drums to call upon the spirits to guide and help them, particularly at the time of the Full Moon.

Fire also brings down the spirits: bunches of wormwood are thrown into these fires. The smoke from these fires calls up helping spirits.

On St Luke's day (18 October) day take a sprig each of marjoram, marigold, thyme and wormwood. Dry them before a fire and rub into a fine powder; simmer in a pot with honey and vinegar and anoint yourself three times saying:

> *'St Luke, St Luke be kind to me*
> *In dreams let my true love be seen.*

Notes

1. The Doctrine of Signatures was an ancient belief that plants resembled the diseases they cured. Thus, heart-shaped leaves for the heart, yellow flowers for the liver, red for the blood . . .

2. Not to be confused with dead nettles which are used for different purposes.

3. Quoted in Marian Woodman, *The Owl was A Baker's Daughter: Obesity, Anorexia Nervosa and the Repressed Feminine.* (See the Bibliography for full details of this book.)

6
HERBS OF SATURN

Element: *Earth*

Organ: *Spleen*

Realm: *Thought*

Humour: *Melancholic*

Function: *Retention*

Qualities: *Hot and dry*

The herbs of Saturn included in this book are: comfrey, horsetail, mullein and shepherd's purse.

Herbs of Saturn balance fluid in the body, make things colder and drier, build up deposits, concentrate and solidify tissues and secretions. They have the quality of binding. Saturn herbs have their actions countered by those of Jupiter most strongly, and to a lesser extent by those of the Sun and Mars. Saturn in its turn opposes the Moon and Venus.

COMFREY

Planetary ruler: Saturn

Qualities: *Cold and dry*

Harvest time:
*leaves and flowers:
June to August,
root: November
to March*

Parts used:
Flowers, leaves and root

Scientific name:
Symphytum officinale

Medical uses:
*For bones,
wounds and
the digestive
system*

Main constituents:
*Allantoin, tannins, gum, resins,
alkaloids,[1] mucilage, B12 in
flowering tops, calcium.*

Myths and legends

Comfrey's medical name, *Symphytum*, comes from the Greek *sympho* meaning to unite which describes its action in knitting bones; indeed, one of its common names is knitbone. Other are: knitback, consound, blackwort, bruisewort, slippery root and ass ear.

Comfrey was traditionally eaten as a vegetable in Ireland and was used as a cure for weak blood.

Physical uses

Herb

The flowering tops of comfrey have been found to contain B12 which is needed by vegans to supplement their diet. The herb has a close affinity with the lungs and kidneys and cools hot, dry inflammations affecting those organs. It is soothing and healing to tissue. Allantoin is another substance also found in the flowers and is believed to be responsible for helping cells to regenerate after damage caused by infection or disease. Thus for any action where cell growth is required, where healing of tissue is needed, use the aerial part of the plant rather than the root. Once a wound is beginning to dry up and close, comfrey can be used to accelerate the healing process.

Saturn rules the skeleton, the skin, ligaments and joints and it follows that a herb of Saturn would heal these areas. Comfrey is the remedy par excellence for healing all skeletal connective and ligamental tissue. Use for sprains, fracture, torn ligaments, crush injuries and non-infected wounds. The herb will heal tissues in record time and prevent the deposition of scar tissue. It is useful for chronic skin disease, especially psoriasis, where its action on the skin cells appears to slow down the rate of growth found in this condition – it regulates the growth of cells, and has a normalising, balancing action, and this nicely illustrates Saturn's action in opposing the rapid cell turnover of Jupiter and putting cell replication back to its normal limits.

Comfrey is of great use in arthritis, particularly when the

disease has changed from being hot and inflammatory to cold and deep-seated.

Root
The root contains a large quantity of mucilage and cools and soothes inflammed tissue, particularly that of the digestive system. Its main use is in hot, dry conditions of the gut, such as dyspepsia (acid indigestion), peptic ulcers and irritable bowel syndrome, where it regulates and calms spasm (opposing the muscle spasm of Mars) and forms a protective coat over the inflammed area to give it time to heal.

Recipe
The following recipe is for women who have heavy periods and who are anaemic and for women who have had many pregnancies and have not eaten well.

For weakness and debility, especially for women of childbearing age (after Dr Coffin)

> A large handful of comfrey root
> 50 g (2 oz) broken ginger roots
> a handful of horehound (*marrubium vulgare*)
> 2 nutmegs
> 1 x 5 ml (1 tea)spoon cayenne pepper
> 1 kg (2 lb) sugar

Mix together the comfrey, ginger and horehound. Boil in unpolluted rain water and add the nutmeg, cayenne and sugar. Simmer and stir until all the sugar is dissolved. Bottle.

Dose: take 1 x 5 ml (table)spoon three to four times daily.

Emotional uses
Comfrey relates to the base chakra, the place where energy is stored, where potential is kept. Being of Saturn and of the element earth and connected with the lower energy centres,

comfrey is helpful for those who lack structure and form in their lives, who need to develop within themselves a solid base from which to start out. Comfrey has an affinity with the darkness of chaos and despair and can help in our time to give some sense and order to the chaos which is felt. As a powerful healer of wounds, comfrey can help to heal emotional traumas, particularly where loss is involved and there is felt to be a raw and sensitive wound in the psyche. Comfrey can provide a soothing and grounding protective layer, while the person heals. The herb is particularly helpful for women for have suffered near-death experiences or grave injury. It slowly helps to build up stamina, working in a spiralling, cyclical fashion and earthing the person back into life.

Drink a tea of comfrey first thing in the morning. Take this for as long as you feel the need.

Magical and ritual uses
Known as Hecuba's bells, comfrey is used in rituals of the dark moon, the crone aspect of the Goddess, where rituals of power and wisdom are used to root aspirations and manifest them in the world. Use for releasing/cutting cords that bind you to another and for empowerment after attack; it has the power to destroy and construct. It is cold, deep with a natural dignity and authority, and is a herb of Hecate, goddess of the night, of wild and wintry places. It is an organiser and transformer and can be used in alchemical work. Mixed with mugwort, it deepens trance and aids concentration in spell work and visualisation.

HORSETAIL

Planetary ruler: *Saturn*

Qualities: *Cold and dry*

Harvest time: *June and July*

Parts used: *Whole plant*

Scientific name:
Equisetum arvense

Medicinal uses:
*For the
bones and blood*

Main constituents:
*Silica, saponins,
flavonoids,
alkaloids,
aluminium,
potassium*

Myths and legends

The name comes from the Latin *equus*, meaning a horse and *seta*, a bristle.

Horsetail was once used to clean pewter and other metals. Its silica content kept them bright.

It is thought that the Romans used the bristles of the plant for healing wounds.

Physical uses

Horsetail builds up bone and other tissue in the body. Silica and other minerals build up deficient blood and increase the amount of calcium, iron and other minerals in the body. So the herb is useful where there has been acute blood loss, as in childbirth, miscarriage or a bad accident, or with chronic anaemia owing to heavy periods, late pregnancy, stomach or duodenal ulcers.

WARNING. Any woman who is an insulin-dependent diabetic should not try to regulate her blood sugar levels with horsetail unless supervised by a medical practitioner.

Taken together with nettle, horsetail can build up haemoglobin levels in record time and so is extremely useful in simple iron deficiency anaemia. Horsetail is also an astringent (as a result of Saturn's coldness and dryness) and will stop bleeding from the lungs, kidneys or digestive system.

Useful in bladder and kidney infections, horsetail opposes the 'sweetness' of Venus, making the urine more acidic which prevents bacteria from flourishing. For the same reason, horsetail is one of the herbs used to regulate sugar balance in the body.

As a bone-builder, horsetail can be useful if it is taken in conjunction with comfrey and nettle where there are brittle bones in post-menopausal women. Here, exercise is most important to bring blood to the skeletal tissue to encourage growth and renewal. Tai Chi or Hatha Yoga are particularly recommended, as these exercises not only tone the muscles

and joints, but also build up the vital spirit and therefore resistance and general vitality.

Taken over a period of months, horsetail will help to build up and repair damaged hair, nails and skin and speed up the healing of broken bones.

Traditionally, horsetail was used for tuberculosis to build up stamina and to strengthen the constitution; the silica helps to rebuild the tensile strength in the lungs.

As an astringent, horsetail is useful in cases of stress incontinence, that is, coughing or sneezing, or prolapse of the womb or bladder to strengthen the muscles of the bladder and uterus. Take internally (by mouth) and use as a douche.

Recipes
A bath for rheumatic pain

Take 30 g (1¼ oz) of dried horsetail and steep in boiling water for one hour. Strain and add to the bathwater. Lie in the water for as long as possible.

A douche for prolapse
   50 g (2 oz) horsetail
   50 g (2 oz) shepherd's purse

Mix together with 1 litre (1¾ pints) of water. Heat and reduce to half the quantity.

Pour into a douche bag and douche once daily, retaining the liquid for as long as possible.

Emotional uses
Horsetail is connected with the root chakra, with foundations, survival and basic structures. It has a cleansing, ordering function.

Drink as a tea, preferably at night, for as long as you feel the need.

As a herb of Saturn, horsetail helps to balance excess of melancholic humour – depression, feeling isolated or unloved – while at the same time it strengthens expression of the constructive elements of the melancholic type (that is, thoughtfulness, concentration, being methodical).

Magical and ritual uses
Samhain ritual – burying the hatchet
Some witches say this festival marks the end of the year and that it is the time to settle old scores and wipe the slate clean, ready for the new year. The ritual is best performed in a group.

Gather outside where you can safely have a small fire. Bring with you a large metal cauldron or cooking-pot. Set it down in the middle. Cast a circle, invoking the four elements and Hecate the dark goddess, who rules hidden, secret things. Each woman takes a piece of paper and writes on it the things she wishes to leave behind which belong to the year that has passed. These may be painful events, people, things they have outgrown, old scores and resentments she no longer wishes to carry around her. As each woman finishes writing, she takes her piece of paper and, lighting it, drops it in the cauldron, saying goodbye to all it contains. When all have finished, close the circle[2] and, before leaving, scatter the ashes to the four winds and walk away without looking behind.

MULLEIN

Planetary ruler: *Saturn*

Qualities: *Cool and moist*

Harvest time: *July and August*

Parts used: *Flowers and leaves*

Scientific name: *Verbascum thapsus*

Medicinal uses: *For the lungs
and ears*

Main constituents: *Mucilage, volatile oil,
saponins, resins, flavonoids,
glycosides*

Myths and legends
Roman women were said to have infused the flowers and
mixed the brew with lye to dye their hair yellow.

Mullein seeds are narcotic and poachers were reputed to
have drugged fish with them to make poaching easier.

The herb has also been called hag's tapers, our lady's
flannel, Jupiter's staff and Our Lady's candle. Witches were
believed to have used it in their incantations. Mullein was
believed to have the power to drive away evil spirits,
particularly if collected when the Sun was in Virgo and the
Moon in Aries.

Ulyses was said to have taken mullein to protect him
from Circe who used it in her magical rituals.

Hildegard of Bingen considered the decoction of mullein
flowers to be specific for hoarseness.

Physical uses
Mullein cools and moistens heat and dryness in the lungs. It
tones the membranes of the lungs, reduces irritation and
has an overall sedative effect. It makes phlegm in the lungs

more liquid, releasing blockages or mucous plugs which are found with asthma and chronic bronchitis. It forms the basis for many proprietory cough mixtures and can be used with confidence for bronchitis, tonsillitis, pleurisy and asthma. Traditionally, it was used in the treatment of tuberculosis, which in part can be said to be a Saturnine disease, the tubercles, or lesions, representing solidification of matter. Mullein was said to reduce the cough and production of excess phlegm. It can be used in whooping cough to relax the spasm of the airways, by opposing Mars and cooling the hot, irritated lungs.

Saturn rules the ears and mullein is *the* herb for all ear problems: earache, tinnitus, mastoid infections, accumulations of wax and any head pain caused by ear problems. Mullein is said to affect the auditory nerve and can be used with other medicines in illnesses affecting the balance mechanism. In my opinion it is unnecessary and potentially dangerous to put medicines in the ear and I would treat all the above by giving mullein to be drunk as a tea or tincture. It works perfectly well taken like this and has the added benefit of being safer.

A conserve of mullein flowers applied externally has been found useful in cases of ringworm and other skin infections.

Recipes
For hayfever

Drink 10 g (¼ oz) mullein in tea mixed with eye bright and 1 x 2.5 ml (½ tea)spoon bee pollen as soon as the mullein leaves appear. Drink daily and continue all summer.

Conserve used for ringworm and erysipelas
Fill a large earthenware pot with 25 g (1 oz) mullein flowers and pour on sufficient honey to cover. Let stand for six weeks, strain and bottle. This mixture can also be used as a cough linctus.

Dose: 1 x 5 ml (1 tea)spoon three to six times daily in warm water.

Mullein oil

>25 g (1 oz) fresh flowers
>600 ml (1 pint) olive oil

Macerate over a low heat and cook until all the moisture is drawn off. Strain and bottle.

Use as a lotion for haemorrhoids and chillblains.

Emotional uses

Mullein is said to rule the brow chakra, connected with psychic and spiritual vision. It is the higher octave of the solar plexus chakra, and a receiving centre of a more refined type. The seat of spiritual will, the brow chakra, is not generally awakened in those who are ruled by their emotions to the exclusion of 'higher' impulses.

When you feel that you are in need of a 'lift', brew a pot of mullein tea, sip slowly and affirm to yourself your divinity and your sacredness.

Magical and ritual uses

The brow chakra is concerned with seeing, the ability to plan and be forwarned. Mullein was used by Amazon warriors to scry for the enemy's battle plans – they used it on crystal balls.

It can be burnt as incense, although it is very smoky so do not use in a confined space. Mixed with mugwort it enhances the development of clairvoyance. Use as a sleep pillow for astral travelling and projection. It will clear a psychic space after work; wash the floor/altar/tools with a tea made from it.

SHEPHERD'S PURSE

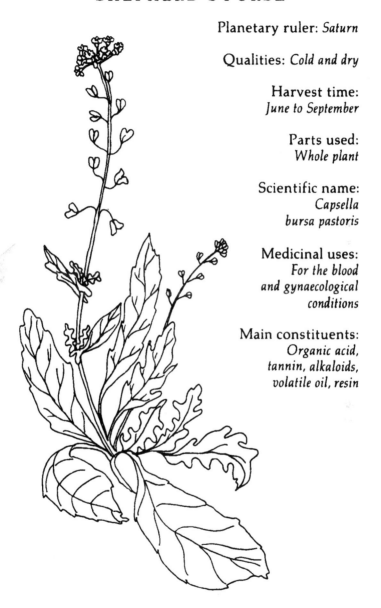

Planetary ruler: *Saturn*

Qualities: *Cold and dry*

Harvest time:
June to September

Parts used:
Whole plant

Scientific name:
*Capsella
bursa pastoris*

Medicinal uses:
*For the blood
and gynaecological
conditions*

Main constituents:
*Organic acid,
tannin, alkaloids,
volatile oil, resin*

Myths and legends
Shepherd's purses were known as witches' pouches. Heart or Diana's arrow heads describe the shape of the seed pods.

Physical uses
Being dry and cold, shepherd's purse clots blood, cools it and therefore staunches haemorrhages, discharges and fluxes such as diarrhoea. It is strong and can be used to oppose heavy bleeding at puberty and the menopause, thereby opposing Venus' expulsive faculty and Jupiter's improper composition of the blood. It will also reduce the muscle spasm of Mars as found in some types of menstrual cramps. It will dry up vaginal secretions (the non-specific kind) and is also useful in a type of thrush where there is redness, heat and itching; it cools and binds together these mucous membranes. Use when excess blood has coagulated and collected in the uterus, for example, with fibroids and endometriosis (a disease of the wound), with an expulsive remedy (that is, a herb of Venus or the Moon) to expel the accumulated humour.

Shepherd's purse is useful where phelgm has accumulated in the bladder or uterus, such as in cystitis where the infection has become deep-seated or gone cold and likewise in any similar urinary tract infection. It has been used with success with bed-wetting children. (In such cases, mix with a little agrimony and give in tincture form, not tea.)

Use the herb fresh in a decoction for diarrhoea and dysentery, first identifying the cause of the diarrhoea. Diarrhoea can be a cleansing process, especially for children, but if allowed to continue for too long the child or adult will begin to dehydrate. Children, through loss of fluids and electrolytes, can die from bowel infections.

Shepherd's purse treats stones in the kidney or bladder. Stones are given to Saturn, as they are concentrated dried material which has accumulated in the body. Generally, stones appear when the body fluids become too concentrated so that solids precipitate and collect in the hollow organs such as the gallbladder, kidneys and the bladder.

WARNING. Shepherd's purse is not to be taken by pregnant women as it has an astringent effect on the uterus. However, women having home deliveries or midwives who use herbs would do well to have tincture of shepherd's purse in their first-aid kit. As a powerful anti-haemorrhagic remedy, it is most useful in cases of larger than normal blood loss after delivery, before this becomes a medical emergency. Fifteen drops in an egg cupful of cold water taken every ten to fifteen minutes will staunch the blood flow quickly and safely. As an astringent, shepherd's purse is useful in uterine prolapse. Use as a douche or take internally over several months.

Shepherd's purse will staunch the bleeding of wounds and nose bleeding. Soak a cotton wool pad of the fresh juice in a little cold water and press on the wound.

Note The potency of dried shepherd's purse declines rapidly, so either use the fresh herb which grows abundantly on most waste ground, or make a tincture from the fresh herb to ensure maximum potency.

Recipe
For cystitis

> 75 g (3 oz) shepherd's purse
> 75 g (3 oz) comfrey
> 75 g (3 oz) thyme
> 600 ml (1 pint) water

Bring to the boil and simmer in a covered saucepan for ten minutes.

Dose: drink during the course of the day. Repeat for up to five days. If the symptoms persist, consult a practitioner.

Emotional uses
Shepherd's purse is a herb of the solar plexus, providing strength and boundaries. It stabilises and grounds, being of the element earth. Use where the solar plexus is too open

and energised, where impressions, sensations and feelings rush in and the woman becomes overwhelmed by sensation and loses her centre. Shepherd's purse develops the will, providing clarity, definition, precision and the ability to work within limitations and boundaries and enables the woman to develop a clear sense of what her own will might be, so that she is less likely to become overwhelmed and become subject to the will of others. For women who are over sensitive and malleable, shepherd's purse gives emotional strength and is refreshing to the spirit.

Drink as a tea whenever you feel the need.

Magical and ritual uses

Like comfrey, shepherd's purse is a herb that works in spirals, penetrating deep within. It has a divinatory quality, allowing the user to get to the heart of matters. It has both a rooting and firming action and also an other worldliness – it is deep and mysterious. It has a connection with Hecate and the festival of Samhain – that is, the connection with other worlds, with death and sorcery, and seeks the mysteries behind the veils of illusion.

Divination

On the Samhain full moon (that is, the full moon nearest to 31 October), take yourself to a secluded spot. Visualise a triangle of white light and sit yourself in the centre. At each point of the triangle, invoke one of the faces of the Goddess: mother, maiden and crone. On a charcoal disc, burn dried shepherd's purse and mugwort. Pour pure spring water into a ceramic bowl and allow the reflection of the Full Moon to be caught in it. Let the water settle. Invoke the fates, courage, wisdom and clarity to be with you in your triangle and call on Hecate, mother of the shades, to part the veil of illusion and let you see how things really stand. When you have seen enough, thank the Goddess and offer the water as a libation to Her wisdom. Dismiss the fates with thanks, visualise the triangle dispersing. Destroy all signs of your presence before leaving where you have been. Walk away without turning back.

Notes

1 There has been evidence to suggest that the alkaloids contained in comfrey can cause liver cancer in experimental animals. I do not think the evidence is conclusive and I am deeply sceptical about, and hostile towards, experiments with laboratory animals. These results are at variance with the traditional use of comfrey for malignancy. I have used comfrey extensively for long periods over the last twelve years with no ill effects.
2 To close a circle, see chapter 2 p 83.

7
HERBS OF MERCURY

Element: *Earth*

Organ: *Lungs and nervous systems*

Realm: *Thought*

Humour: *Melancholic*

Function: *Retention*

The herbs of Mercury work on the nervous system and the lungs, both ruled by this planet. They will ground, stabilise and sedate the person. As they are melancholic remedies, herbs of Mercury generally have a slight depressant quality about them, useful in anxiety where the nervous system is over-stimulated, but to be used with caution with those who are depressed.

The herbs of mercury included in this book are: elecampane, fennel, lavender, liquorice and valerian.

ELECAMPANE

Planetary ruler: *Mercury*

Qualities: *Hot and dry*

Harvest time: *November to March*

Parts used: *Root (in the second year and better fresh)*

Scientific name: *Inula Helenium*

Medicinal use: *For the lungs*

Main constituents: *Volatile oil, bitters, triterpenes, mucilage, inulin*

Myths and legends

Helenium is said to refer to Helen; the plant was said to have sprung from where her tears fell on the ground when Paris kidnapped her.

Galen and Hippocrates[1] both used the plant for its beneficial effect on the womb, the urinary system and the lungs.

In Denmark elecampane is called elf dock.

Elecampane is often mentioned in mediaeval herbals; it was called *marchalan* by thirteenth-century Welsh physicians.

A Latin ditty runs: 'Enula campana reddit praecordia sana.' ('Elecampane will sustain the spirits.')

Physical uses

Although a herb of Mercury, elecampane is very hot and dry and so needs to be used with care so as not to precipitate a fever. Use with chronic catarrh (phlegmatic illnesses opposing Moon and Venus), acute catarrhal asthma, whooping cough and bronchitis with copious phlegm.

191

Elecampane is warming and strenthening to lung tissue, a stimulating expectorant useful for a debilitating cough, especially where there is a strong, nervous element to the condition, as Mercury rules the nerves. Elecampane detoxifies the lungs and promotes the healing of tissue. Use in small doses in the treatment of chronic lung conditions such as pneumoconiosis (miners' lung), and emphysema, with soothing remedies.

Elecampane reduces inflammation and clears infectious disease. It induces sweating and lowers the temperature. Use for coughs which are bad at night and when lying down.

WARNING. Because of its heat, use very sparingly, if at all, for choleric and sanguine types.

Recipes
Elecampane Wine

Steep 75 g (3 oz) of root in 1 litre (1¾ pints) of red wine for ten days. Shake the bottle frequently. Strain and add honey to taste.

Dose: I wineglass twice daily; to stimulate the appetite. This mixture also acts as a stomach tonic and cough remedy.

Elecampane Syrup (after Culpeper)
'The fresh roots of Elecampane preserved with sugar or made into a conserve, or a syrup, are very effectual to warm a cold windy stomach and stitches in the side, caused by the spleen and to relieve coughs, shortness of breath and wheezing of the lungs.'

Soothing tea for bronchitis
Equal parts of elecampane root, thyme, nettle and lungwort.

Steep 1 x 5 ml (1 tea)spoon in ½ cup of boiling water two to three times daily.

Emotional uses

Elecampane is related to the brow chakra and the use of the 'higher mind'. It is useful for intellectuals, people who live in their heads and as a result are cut off from their physical bodies. Such people usually have thin, boney, ill-cared for physical forms and are often rigid emotionally.

Elecampane gently helps to unblock this very stuck material and allows the person to breathe emotionally again, to relax a little and trust her feelings more.

Take 5 drops of the tincture daily for as long a you feel the need.

Magical and ritual uses

The brow chakra is connected with clairvoyance, the ability to see clearly, to be able to use the mind as a tool, to create thought forms. It wills things to happen, using spiritual will rather than the emotional will of the solar plexus. Thus the energy of the brow chakra is neutral, non-attached and has no emotion connected with it.

Meditation on clarity

When the moon is in an air or earth sign, late in the evening take yourself off to a quiet place where you will be left undisturbed for fifteen minutes. Light three candles, one white, one blue and one yellow. On a disc of charcoal, sprinkle dried elecampane and allow the space to fill up with the smoke. Close your eyes and focus your attention on the spot between your eyebrows. Take a few deep breaths and be aware that a beam of light is coming from that place. It will shine on areas in your life which need clarifying. Allow images and feelings to come up and try not to analyse or reject anything. Take as long as it feels appropriate for you to explore, and when you feel ready, slowly come back into the room. Take some time to write down your experiences. You may need to do this meditation several times over a period of weeks.

The will

There are three types: strong will, skilful will and transpersonal will. The one we are familiar with is the strong will of our Victorian past, where we are forced against our will to do unpleasant things to 'develop our characters'. Skilful will needs to be developed by all of us. It is the will which manoevres, like a woman undertaking a martial art, using the strength or force of her opponent to overcome her antagonist, being poised and balanced, ready to move in any direction as the need arises, manipulating the forces of nature appropriate to the task in hand. Transpersonal will is to do with the laws of Karma, the will of the Goddess – whatever forces there are that direct and inform one's soul in its incarnation. A woman can choose to live in accordance with transpersonal will, whatever that might mean for her. Or she may choose to go against the sense of rightness and operate from her personal desires and, in effect, make no progress in her life. (See *The Act of Will*, by Roberto Assagioli and *What We May Be* by Piero Ferrucci.)

Connecting with the transpersonal will

Take yourself to a quiet place where you will be undisturbed for at least forty-five minutes. Sit comfortably and relax your body. Take a few deep breaths to relax yourself, breathing out the tensions of the day. Close your eyes and imagine you are in a meadow on a sunny day. Look around you, see the plants growing, feel the warm sun on you, be aware of any animals or insects in the vicinity. Really be in this meadow. Walk around and explore a little. Shortly you will see a path leading from the meadow. Follow this path as it leads up a mountain side. As you walk, look at the surrounding countryside as you slowly make your ascent. Gradually the air becomes clearer as you near the summit of the mountain. As you move closer to the top you become aware of a stillness, a magical quality which surrounds you. Finally you reach the top. There is an archway, and passing through this you see a fountain. Walk towards the fountain and notice your surroundings. You become aware of a beam of light shining down from the sun into the water of the fountain. Travelling along this beam of light is a symbol of your transpersonal will. It may be a person, an animal, an object or even a sound or colour. Whatever it is, allow the symbol to come near to you. This symbol has a message for you about your transpersonal will. Take some time to ask questions or listen to what it has to say to you . . .

When you feel you have learned enough, take your leave of the symbol. Before you go you will be given a gift to remind you of this meeting. Slowly make your way down the mountain back into the meadow. When you are ready, open your eyes and write down what happened to you.

FENNEL

Planetary ruler: *Mercury*

Qualities: *Hot and dry*

Harvest time: *Autumn*

Parts used: *Seeds*

Scientific name: *Foeniculum vulgare*

Medicinal use: *For the digestive
system*

Main constituents: *Volatile oil*

Myths and legends
The poet Longfellow wrote of the virtue of the plant

> *Above the lower plants it towers*
> *The Fennel with its yellow flowers*
> *And in an earlier age than ours*
> *Was gifted with the wondrous powers*
> *Lost vision to restore.*

Fennel is linked with milk and lactating. The cow was a very common manifestation of the Great Mother; white, milk giving, sustaining, nourishing mother of all. In Egypt she was revered as Hathor whose udder produced the Milky Way, and who daily gave birth to the Sun. Early myths show the universe being curdled into shape from the milk of a cow. In India there is a Creation myth known as the 'Churning of the Sea of Milk'. The Egyptian goddess as birth-giver was depicted as having a cow's head with horns and two breasts. She gave each Eygptian a secret soul name (*ren*), and was called Renenet, the Lady of the Double Granary, whose nourishment was inexaustible.

Physical uses

Mercury in Virgo opposes Pisces and so fennel expels the
phlegmatic humour. Being hot and dry, it gets rid of cold
and dampness. It calms flatulence and helps to expel wind
from the body.

A tea of fennel seeds, drunk in the last few days of
pregnancy and when breastfeeding, will increase milk
production in the mother and pass through her milk to the
baby, helping to reduce any wind colic. As a volatile oil,
fennel stiumates digestion, helps reduce bloating after
meals and sluggish digestion. It increases the appetite for
those who have lost their taste for food. Culpeper says it:
'. . . help to open obstructions of the liver, spleen, and gall,
and thereby ease the painful and windy swellings of the
spleen.'

Fennel is also a lung remedy. It soothes harsh, irritating
coughs and helps to rid the airways of phlegm. It is useful in
bronchitis, asthma or any lung condition where there is an
accumulation of catarrh.

The juice of the plant has a long tradition of being helpful
to the eyesight; dropped into the eyes it will clear mistiness
and any infection.

Recipes
Soothing eye bath

Mix together 1 x 2.5 ml (½ tea)spoon each of eyebright,
chamomile and fennel. Add to 1 cup of boiling water and let
stand, covered. Use cool and strained.

Trotula's recipe for menstrual pain

Mix together juniper berries, parsley, fennel, rock parsely,
lovage and catnip with wine. Drink warm.

Emotional uses

Fennel is nourishing and sustaining, like mother's milk. It
has a calming, soothing effect, for those who are soft,
docile, gentle, quiet people. It helps to open up those who

have been frightened or starved of love and nourishment. It is for anorexics, over-eaters, those who cannot nourish and take care of themselves but look for 'mother figures' to do it for them. The herb helps to loosen fears over sensuality, and opens the person up to the delights of the body.

For this reason fennel is excellent for new mothers, to help build up the bond between mother and child and to allow for mutual nourishment.

Drink the tea whenever you feel you are in need of nourishment.

Magical and ritual uses
To celebrate the birth of a child
At the first opportunity, and before forty-one days have passed after the birth, meet together with mothers and children. Each woman should bring something for the new mother, preferably something handmade or sweet smelling, but definitely not practical – something she can adorn herself with.

Fennel was traditionally brought for new mothers, bunches to be hung near the cradle to keep away the flies, and to be drunk as a tea to help the flow of milk. Green is the colour of the heart, of fertility and birth. Welcome the woman into this new stage of life.

LAVENDER

Planetary ruler: *Mercury*

Qualities: *Hot and dry*

Harvest time: *June to August*

Parts used: *Flowers*

Scientific name: *Lavendula officinalis*

Medicinal use: *For nervous disorders*

Main constituents: *Volatile oil, tannin, bitters*

Myths and legends

Lavender's name comes from the Latin *lavare* to wash.

Lavender was dedicated to Hecate, Media and Circe and was used to avert the Evil Eye.

Witches call lavender elf leaf.

Lavender was said to have been an ingredient of the Four Thieves Vinegar, said to have been used by grave robbers during the great plagues, to prevent them from catching the disease.

Lavender and rosemary worn together were said to preserve chastity.

Physical uses

Lavender as a herb of Mercury in Gemini is a remedy for the nervous system. It is as strong as valerian but does not have its serious side effects or addictive possibilities. Use Lavender for insomnia where there is physical tension or a mind which cannot slow down and stop thinking, for women who work with their intellect and find it difficult to 'wind down' at the end of the day. Conversely, use for those whose minds are not receiving enough stimulation during the day and are still 'awake' at night. Take lavender tea thirty minutes before retiring, or rub the essential oil around the temples and put a few drops on the pillow before getting into bed.

WARNING. Lavender can be used to wean people off addictive substances. It is most important, however, for anyone who has taken benzodiazapenes (such as Valium) or tranquillisers *not* to suddenly stop taking these drugs, because a severe withdrawal reaction might be precipitated. Instead, cut the dose down gradually, under the watchful eye of a physician, complementary or orthodox.

Lavender is one of the best remedies for the treatment of migraine, both to curb an attack and for the long-term treatment of the ailment. To stop an attack, draw a hot bath and drop 15-20 drops of essential oil of lavender into it. Lie still in the bath for fifteen to twenty minutes, keeping the water hot. Then lie in a darkened room. You will probably sleep for a while, and when you wake the pain will have gone.

Lavender is also useful for dizzyness and faintness, travel and sea sickness. Take as a tincture or inhale lavender water from a handkerchief.

Lavender acts as a digestive stimulant. It acts on the liver, clearing stagnation due to excess blood; it strengthens the stomach and reduces bloating after meals, wind, distension and poor absorption of food.

Lavender lowers the blood pressure and calms palpitations of the heart and hot flushes.

The herb is a powerful antiseptic and can be used both internally and externally for infections and infestations. It cleanses the blood stream of toxins and resists poisons and insect bites. Lavender can be used as a gargle under supervision for tonsillitis and sore throats, for infected gums and mouth ulcers, and for toothache.

The essential oil has been used to treat burns, diluted in almond or olive oil: 1 part lavender to 10 parts oil.

WARNING. Do not use lavender if using insulin for diabetes.

Recipe
Migraine
Mix equal parts of rosemary and lavender. Make tea in the usual way and drink daily for at least four weeks to balance the circulation of blood to the brain.

Emotional uses
Lavender is a herb of the solar plexus which resides above the navel, and as such is concerned with the assimilation of external stimuli. The solar plexus is like a receiving dish; if uncontrolled, it will pick up whatever vibrations, feelings and emotions are in the atmosphere and react to those sensations in an instinctive way – that is, a 'gut' reaction. Most people function primarily through this chakra and many are in a sense at its mercy because, until the head and heart centres are operating, they are ruled by their desires and cannot use detachment or objectivity to modify their responses. It is said that, as a race, we are in the process of moving our focus from the solar plexus to the heart chakra and we are therefore becoming less self-centred and more group-orientated. (See Alice Bailey, *The Soul and Its Mechanism*) Lavender acts as a filter to the solar plexus to block some of these stimuli and enables the woman to begin to discriminate about the sensory material she chooses to absorb. With awareness, it is possible to close down this chakra for protection and absorb only those impulses which are healthful and nourishing. The more tuned a woman becomes to her environment, the more awareness she has of how violence, greed and ugliness disturb her internal equilibrium. The aim is not to become a sensitive, rarified plant which cannot function in the world, but rather a discriminating individual who chooses not to associate with the cruder, coarser aspects of life.

Put 5 drops of the essential oil in a bath and lie in this, breathing in its scent and letting go of feeling you want to lose.

Magical and ritual uses
Lavender flowers were thrown on midsummer fires to bring visions and inspiration to the witches. Inhaling the smoke of burning lavender induces a trance state; it brings clarity and coherence to pathworkings and is excellent for focusing the mind on a particular task. It is for creating images of how you wish an event to unfold, and for imaging.

Lavender ritual
Lavender, collected in the summer months to be used in the following spring, is a herb of the spring equinox – the early morning, the new moon – and represents the first shafts of sunlight that herald winter's end, the beginning of journeys, the start of new ventures. Early morning meditations when the world is still and new, fresh with the promise of the day and still lingering in some of the mystery of the night. The herb is subtle, delicate, quixotic, Mercurial, and has the essence of blessed beginnings, of potential, of ideas not yet born, of webs yet to be woven and spells spun. Use lavender at the beginning of a venture, with work on the New Moon, for the start of something, especially if it involves travel over water and for intangible ideas. Welcome spring in with lavender fires or with its essence sprinkled in water and used to wash sacred space and magical tools. Likewise welcome a new soul into the world with lavender water and a lavender bag in the crib to keep away snakes and evil omens. And in her ritual bath, bless the mother in her new aspect of womanhood.

LIQUORICE

Planetary ruler: *Mercury*

Qualities: *Hot and moist*

Harvest time: *Autumn*

Parts used: *Root*

Scientific name: *Glycyrrhiza glabra*

Medicinal uses: *For the lungs and*
adrenal system

Main constituents: *Mucilage, flavonid glycosides,*
including glycyrrhzin,
steroidal saponins, glucose,
bitters, oestrogenic substances,
coumarins

Myths and legends

Glukos is Greek for sweet and *riza* is also Greek meaning a root.

Liquorice was called scythic, named after the scythian soldiers who were reputed to be able to survive for ten days without eating or drinking by chewing liquorice root.

St Hildegard recommended using liquorice to cleanse the lungs and clear the voice.

Physical uses

Liquorice is anti-inflammatory and anti-rheumatic; it has a steroidal-like action and is used for chronic inflammatory conditions such as arthritis, asthma, peptic ulcer and Addison's disease. Liquorice reduces the acidity of the stomach and provides a thick layer of mucilage which protects the lining of the digestive and respiratory tracts to allow for healing to occur. Working on the liver, liquorice increases bile excretion. It relaxes spasm of smooth muscle in the gut and respiratory system.

Liquorice reduces fever and lowers blood cholesterol levels.

WARNING. It has been suggested that liquorice can raise blood pressure, so watch carefully if there has been a history of high blood pressure.

Liquorice is the primary remedy in most herbal cough medicines, and is used by herbalists to sweeten bitter tasting mixtures. It soothes a dry, irritating cough.

Liquorice has been called the female equivalent of ginseng. Like ginseng it is an adaptogen, a substance which increases the action of chemicals in the body: vitamins, minerals, hormones and any drugs, medicinal or otherwise. Both ginseng and liquorice work on the adrenal glands, increasing stamina, stimulating the body's defence mechanisms and helping the body to resist stress. Ginseng is stimulating, whereas liquorice is harmonising. The root is an especially useful adjunct to hormonal treatment in women, the absence of menstruation, problems at puberty and menopause, infertility or miscarriage. It builds the stamina of the woman, increasing her life-force so that she is able to cope with the stresses brought about by these conditions.

WARNING. Liquorice taken over a long period of time may deplete the body of potassium. To avoid this, take dandelion herb to boost the level of potassium in the body.

Recipes
A Cough Syrup

> 1 x 5 ml (tea) spoon linseed
> 25 g (1 oz) liquorice root
> 100 g (4 oz) raisins
> 100 g (4 oz) brown sugar
> 1 x 15 ml (table) spoon vinegar

Simmer the first four ingredients down to 1 quart. Add the sugar and vinegar.

Drink 300 ml ($\frac{1}{2}$ pint) of the mixture before going to bed.

Mouthwash

    30 g ($1\frac{1}{4}$ oz) dried liquorice root
    500 ml (18 fl oz) water

Bring to the boil and simmer for fifteen minutes.

Use for red and inflammed mouth, tongue and gums.

Tea for bronchitis

Use equal parts of anise, liquorice, plantain, fennel seeds and coltsfoot leaves.

Mix 1 x 5 ml (tea)spoon of the mixture in $\frac{1}{2}$ cup boiling water.

Bring to the boil and sweeten to taste. Take three cups daily.

For measles

    4 parts safflowers
    4 parts melissa
    2 parts liquorice
    2 parts elderflowers
    1 part violet leaves

Boil 1 x 5 ml (tea)spoon of the mixture in three cups of water for three minutes; let stand for ten minutes. Take one cup three times daily.

A drink called 'cure all' was a mixture of liquorice, couchgrass and barley.

Emotional uses

Liquorice is a dark and mysterious root. It is connected with the passions: love, hate, lust, revenge, madness and rage. The shadow side where the instincts have free reign, where

205

madness lives. The madness born of sexual passion, obsession, raw instinctual energies. Its power is dark and hidden, not easily accessible.

Drink the tea whenever you feel the need.

Liquorice has the quality of splitting assunder, separating mind from feelings and feelings from physicality. Liquorice relates to the base chakra, the Kundalini fire which can be roused by extremes of emotion, the serpent which destroys and creates. The harnessing of sexual power for creativity or healing. Use where sexual passion is overwhelming people, where they feel out of control with jealousy, hatred or lust. Or where they are frozen and afraid of these powerful, transformative emotions. Because of the strong feelings it can generate it is best not to give liquorice to women who are timid and excessively fearful, who may not be able to contain this kind of energy.

Magical and ritual uses

Kali Ma was the Hindu triple goddess of creation, preservation and destruction. She is generally known in her destroyer aspect, as she devours the entrails of Shiva her mate, while her yoni (vagina) sexually destroys his penis. It is said of her that 'by feeling She is known. How then can lack of feeling find Her?' (From Barbara Walker, *The Woman's Encyclopedia of Myths and Secrets*, p. 490).

Kali is sometimes depicted with a cobra around her waist, suggesting the power and deadliness of the womb, and how motherhood is closely tied to death.

Tantricism is the system of Yoni workship, the veneration of woman-centred sexuality. It was founded by a secret sect of women in India, thousands of years ago. The sect believed women had more spirituality than men, and that a man could only contact his higher spiritual potential through union with a woman. Through intercourse without ejaculation, men were able to store up their vital fluids; they were believed to absorb the fluid secreted by the woman during her orgasm and store it in the spine. Eventually this fluid would work its way up the chakras to the crown where it would flower forth in divine inspiration.

This belief was in conflict with the Christian and Buddhist beliefs that men should keep away from women as a corrupting and depleting force. In the Tao, the Chinese version of Tantricism, men were also taught to stop ejaculation so as not to deplete their vital energies, and to let their weaker yang nature absorb the yin of a woman's orgasm. Men were counselled to keep this secret as they feared that if women were to supress their orgasms while bringing a man to ecstasy, they would overtake the men in wisdom and energy. The greater yin would stay in their bodies and they would absorb the yang energy of the male.

VALERIAN

Planetary ruler: *Mercury*

Qualities: *Hot and moist*

Harvest time: *November to March*

Parts used: *Root*

Scientific name: *Valeriana officinalis*

Medicinal use: *For nervous conditions*

Main constituents: *Volatile alkaloids, volatile oil (which contains valerianic acid)*

Myths and legends

Valeriana comes from the Latin *valere*, meaning to be powerful. It also means to be in health.

Valerian was supposed to inspire love and was used in love philtres. It was said that if a woman wore valerian, she would never lack lovers. (This seems unlikely because of the rank smell it gives off!)

The herb was said to preserve the wearer from both lightning and witchcraft, and to be an antidote for spells.

The Pied Piper was believed to have had valerian hidden in his pockets and that it was this smell that made the rats leave with him. It is true that both rats and cats adore valerian, so store with care or your cat will eat your supply! They have been known to open jars and tear bags apart which contain valerian. A witch's name for valerian is cat's paw.

American Indians use valerian for the treatment of epilespy and for massage with paralysed limbs.

As a sedative for the higher nerve centres, valerian was used to treat shell-shock in the Second World War. The oil of valerian was used in Europe in the treatment of cholera. Culpeper recommends the root for plague.

Physical uses

Valerian is one of the more powerful remedies for the nervous system. As a herb of Mercury, it acts as a sedative and is hypnotic, antispasmodic (opposing Mars), a pain-killer and narcotic. Use in any chronic or severe condition where the whole system needs to be relaxed: chronic anxiety, chronic insomnia, migraines, panic attacks, palpitations, convulsions, *petit mal* and vertigo. Use for women coming off any addictive substance, especially tranquillisers and barbiturates, alcohol and hard drugs. By carefully regulating the dose, withdrawal symptoms can be minimised and some rest achieved.

WARNING. Valerian can be abused and if taken above the recommended dose it has the following effects: headache, mental excitement, hallucination, giddiness, aggitation and spasms.

Use wherever there is severe pain, such as rheumatism and arthritis, kidney stones, neuralgia and shingles. Taken in warm water for severe menstrual cramps, terror in childbirth, miscarriage, and any shock, trauma or accident. In the treatment of pain, by far the best method is to find out the cause of the pain and treat that, and then the pain will disappear. This is not always possible, however, as pains can be sudden and debilitating and certain conditions respond only slowly to treatment. In such instances, judicious use of valerian will ease suffering temporarily while the cause of the pain is being treated more holistically.

Recipes

For irritating coughs

15 g (½ oz) valerian
15 g (½ oz) raisins

15 g (½ oz) aniseed
15 g (½ oz) liquorice

Boil together. Sip with honey.

For shock
5 to 7 drops of valerian tincture in a cupful of warm water.

Neuralgia linament
Add 8 to 12 drops of valerian tincture to 100 g (4 oz) of cold pressed oil and rub in.

Emotional uses

Valerian helps to work with fear which blocks creativity and self-expression. It is for people who are overwhelmed by fear, terrified and unable to move, who may take mood-altering drugs to cope with their panic. Usually they are paralysed by their own thoughts as the fearful object in almost all cases does not exist in the external reality; it is free-floating anxiety rather than fear of tigers on the streets. Once on such a frightened plane, a woman can become an attractive force for any fear in the atmosphere. She becomes bombarded with fear and loses the sense of her own power and courage to such a degree that she cannot draw boundaries between her own emotions and what she is picking up in the general atmosphere. If prolonged, this can lead to madness, as a total loss of self is experienced. Alcohol, tranquillisers, barbiturates and food may be taken in an attempt to ground her feelings and this they may do initially, but ultimately lead to greater disorientation and fear, and the problem will be compounded. Small amounts of valerian calms the emotional body. It gives courage and stamina to the woman and helps to balance the mind and the emotions, bringing some harmony between the two. Over time, it can help to move energy from the solar plexus to the heart, moving the emotions to a higher, more refined space.

WARNING. As it can become addictive, valerian should be taken in small doses, three days on, three days off, to prevent dependency.

By helping to balance the light and dark aspects of the psyche, valerian can reduce the terror of the unconscious, the fear of ghosts, haunting, psychic phenomena, and night terrors. It allows for the person to see a truer reflection of herself: light and shadow, seeing and reconciling, accepting and integrating. Use where there is fear of darkness, of evil powers, demons and vague fears.

Fill a small cotton bag with valerian and sleep with this under your pillow.

Magical and ritual uses
Drink valerian for magical work, going deep into yourself for reincarnation work, magic mirrors, scrying and any dark moon Hecate rituals. A Samhain herb, it helps witches to penetrate deep into the mysteries and to go beyond their normal limits, to deal with fears of loss of self and boundaries. It is used for work on one's dark aspect, the shadow, hag or crone. Returns are accomplished with valerian and any work which repels evil. It is for crossing the styx, the river which divides the living from the dead.

Reincarnation work
Use in a safe place, at night, where you will not be disturbed for at least thrity minutes. Allow yourself to get physically comfortable. Focus your consciousness in that place and breathe deeply a couple of times. Feel yourself rising up, floating up from where you are lying; see your body lying beneath you; allow yourself to travel through the ceiling, through the roof and up, up into space. Stay in space a while, feeling communion with the stars, feeling the vastness of space. Then slowly allow yourself to float downwards, towards earth, and when you land, you will be in another time and place. Allow yourself to explore this place, knowing that you are able to come back at any time you choose. After ten to fifteen minutes, slowly rise up

again in to space. Spend some time here 'clearing yourself' of this experience and then slowly come back to the room and into your body once more.

Notes

1 Hippocrates, born in 460 BC on the island of Cos in Greece, wrote about and practised medicine. His theories were utilised for over 800 years, and doctors to this day adhere to the Hippocratic Oath regarding medical practice and ethics.

PART 3

PRACTICAL
INFORMATION

Collection of herbs

It is quite possible, even for those who live in cities, to collect their own herbs. Most of the common herbs can be found within waste ground, in city gardens and parks and in the commons and marsh lands. Also beside canals and rivers, and in the gardens of deserted houses.

One of the best patches of lady's mantle I have found in London grows in the flower beds of the Royal College of Physicians in Regent's Park. Is this a joke of the Goddess? Is She secretly undermining their patriarchal machinations, or was the gardener a witch? Whatever the reason, it always gladdens my heart when I walk there and I re-affirm to myself that She cannot be defeated.

People are often surprised that I collect my herbs from a city, arguing that pollution from traffic and factories must diminish their value or make them toxic. But everywhere is polluted to a greater or lesser degree. In large cities there is lead pollution, but in rural areas there is the pollution of pesticides which are often sprayed from the air and may be blown on to non-agricultural land and into streams and rivers. Plants absorb these poisons through their circulatory systems. Ever increased radioactivity from nuclear power stations enters the atmosphere and affects all life, including plants. Although we can take precautions to make sure our bodies are not overloaded with toxic chemicals, by eating natural foods and organic vegetables and eschewing chemical medicines, we cannot ensure that our foods and medicines are not physically tainted.

I use herbs that grow in London as this is the place in which I live and work. I see this as taking a homeopathic dose of my environment and hold that it will build up my resistance to environmental pollution. In addition to this, as far as possible I follow the macrobiotic principles of eating, using the things which grow around me so as to be in harmony with my environment.

Collect flowers and leaves in the summer months. Any plant is at its most powerful when the flowers are just about to open, this is when its life force is at its highest. Roots are collected in November, when the sap has descended for the winter, or in March, just before it rises again. If you are astrologically in tune, pick the aerial parts of herbs on a Moon waxing to full, and roots on a waning Moon. Collect herbs on the day represented by their ruling planet: sun plants on a Sunday, Moon plants on a Monday, Mars plants on a Tuesday, Mercury plants on a Wednesday, Jupiter plants on a Thursday, Venus plants on a Friday and Saturn plants on a Saturday.

Real enthusiasts can elect a judicial time for picking by drawing up a chart for the most auspicious time. To maximise their properties, collect them during their planetary hour. The planetary hour begins at dawn. The first hour in any day is ruled by the same planet which rules the day. For example, on Monday, which is ruled by the Moon, the first hour is also ruled by the Moon. The planets then follow in this order: Moon, Mercury, Venus, Mars, Jupiter, Saturn, Sun. To find out the time of sunrise, look in the papers. If this is not possible, because of bad weather, then pick them on a day when the planetary force is compatable, that is, Moon days for Venus plants, Saturn days for Mercury, etc.

Choose your plants carefully: pick only the most healthy and choose herbs which are growing in large clumps (which means that the soil conditions are ideal for the plants). Don't uproot the plant unless you need the root. Quite apart from this being a thoughtless and uncaring act it may also be illegal. Take care to leave some of the plant to propagate next year, and for the next herbalist who comes along.

I like to make an invocation and blessing, thanking the plant for its life and stating my intentions for harvesting it.

'Earth, divine goddess, Mother nature who generatest all things and bringest forth anew the sun which thou hast given to the nations; Guardian of sky and sea and of all gods and powers and through thy power all nature falls silent and then sinks in sleep. And again thou bringest back the light and chasest away night and yet again thou coverest us most securely with thy shades. Thou dost contain chaos infinite, yea and winds and showers and storms; thou sendest them out when thou wilt and causest the seas to roar; thou chases away the sun and arousest the storm. Again when thou wilt thou sendest forth the joyous day and givest the nourishment of life with thy eternal surety; and when the soul departs to thee we return. Thou indeed art duly called great Mother of the gods; thou conquerest by thy divine name. Thou art the source of the strength of nations and of gods, without thee nothing can be brought to perfection or be born; thou art great queen of the gods. Goddess! I adore thee as divine; I call upon thy name; be pleased to grant that which I ask thee, so shall I give thanks to thee, Goddess, with one faith.

'Hear, I beseech thee, and be favourable to my prayer. Whatsover herb thy power dost produce, give, I pray, with goodwill to all nations, to save them and grant me this my medicine. Come to me with thy powers, and howsoever I may use them that they have good success and to whomsoever I may give them. Whatever thou dost grant it may prosper. To thee all things return. To those who rightly receive these herbs from me, do thou make them whole. Goddess, I beseech thee; I pray thee as a suppliant that by thy majesty thou grant this to me.

'Now I make intercession to you all ye powers and herbs and to your majesty, ye whom Earth parent of all hath produced and given you as medicine of health to all nations

and hath put majesty upon you, be, I pray you, the greatest help to the human race. This I pray and beseech from you, and be present here with your virtues, for she who created you hath herself promised that I may gather you into the goodwill of him on whom the art of medicine was bestowed, and grant for health's sake good medicine by grace of your powers. I pray grant me through your virtues that what-soever is wrought by me through you may in all its powers have a good and speedy effect and good success and that I may always be permitted with the favour of your majesty to gather you into my hands and to glean your fruits. So I shall give name to the majesty which ordained your birth.'
(From *The Old English Herbals*, by E.S. Rohde p. 41.)

If you are going to collect a number of herbs, be sure to label or in some way identify them, as it is quite hard to tell dried herbs apart. Collect them in a wicker basket or paper bag, but not in anything plastic, otherwise they will begin to ferment in the heat and may later go mouldy.

I have always felt that one of the nice things about being a herbalist is that you have a wonderful excuse to go about picking flowers on sunny days and exploring the land around you.

Collecting roots is not always such a pleasant pursuit as the weather in autumn and spring often leaves much to be desired – at least in the UK. The roots are dug and washed clean of any soil and cut into half-inch pieces for drying. Plants may also be washed after picking and the following mixture is said to reduce the effects of pollution: Mix 1 cup of cider vinegar with 3.5 litres (1 gallon) of water. Rinse the plants in this mixture. Do not soak the plants as many of their properties are soluble in water.

Drying herbs
Bunches of herbs are best dried hanging up or spread out on trays lined with paper. The plants need plenty of circulating air to dry them thoroughly and to prevent them from going mouldy. I tie the herbs in small bunches and then attach them to coat hangers; this way, many plants can be hung

from the same hanger. Dry them in a sheltered place, away from direct sunlight - a dry cupboard, attic or garden shed will do. Be sure to label everything. They will usually take six to eight weeks to dry thoroughly. To test how dry they are, break a stem of a herb in half, if it breaks cleanly, without any fibres remaining, it is dry.

Do not hang the herbs in the kitchen as fats from cooking will stick to them as they dry, making an unpleasant concoction.

Storage of herbs

Direct sunlight reduces the properties of most plants so any method of storage means keeping them away from the sun. Store the herbs in paper, wood or glass. Do not use plastic as plants react with the chemicals in this material. Glass jars in a cupboard or shady spot are probably the best, but paper bags will suffice as long as they are kept away from damp.

The aerial parts of dried herbs will last for one to two years, and the roots slightly longer. To tell the freshness of a herb sample, look, smell and taste it; the aromatics, for example, (those with volatile oils) should look bright, smell strongly and have a definite taste. Anything which tastes musty or looks pale and sun-bleached has probably been incorrectly stored or kept for too long.

Preparation of herbs

First it has to be said that recommended dosages do seem to vary widely and that this may create confusion in the reader's mind, especially if she has read a number of herbals. Almost all recommended doses are 'correct', however, and the reader should choose the dosage which she herself finds most agreeable. The dosages I use are the result of both working with the herbs I use and as a result of feedback from patients. The dosages work for me but they may not work for you. So experiment, and realise that the less you need to take the better; large doses do not necessarily work better than low ones. In my experience the reverse is true as subtler energies are released in low doses. It is hard to overdose with herbs unless the herbs used are poisonous. With common herbs, if you take too much the only side effects will be a stomach ache, possibly diarrhoea and/or a headache.

Types of remedy

Tisanes

It is best to take a remedy in the form of a tisane, that is, a herbal tea or infusion, as the plant is at its most active and potent in this form. A tisane is, however, less appropriate for children, who will often refuse to take bitter tasting herbs, or for long-term treatment.

I have a special tea pot I use for herbal teas, and when preparing them for myself I make this into a ritual as far as possible; preparing and drinking the tea is a self-affirming process, a way of taking control of your life and health and a time each day when you focus on yourself and your own healing. It is a powerful ritual if done with thoughtfulness.

I use a large handful of the particular herb to be used, say 15 g (½ oz) to about 600 ml (1 pint) of boiling water. Pour the water on the herb and then cover carefully to stop any steam escaping. Let this stand for at least ten minutes and drink a cupful three times a day unless otherwise indicated. If you want you can gently reheat the liquid, but be careful not to boil it, or you can drink it when it has cooled down. A tea made in this way will last two to three days in the fridge. If it is an emergency or you wish to make an extra strong brew, you can put the same quantities in cold water and bring to the boil. Simmer for ten minutes and then stand for a further ten minutes, covered. Most herbs are taken before meals, usually about thirty minutes before; some are taken at bedtime.

Decoctions

A decoction is like a tisane, only stronger, and to be ingested. To make a decoction, use, say, 15 g (½ oz) of the herb to about a pint of water.

There are two ways to make a decoction. The first is by

using cold water. This is for herbs such as comfrey which contain a lot of mucilage, as boiling water would destroy this constituent. Pour cold water on to the herb and let it stand overnight. By morning, the mixture will have a jelly-like consistency. For herbs which do not contain mucilage, put the herb into cold water, bring to the boil and simmer, covered, for ten minutes. (This method is especially useful for twigs and roots; be sure to chop the root or at least bruise it if it is too hard to chop.)

Drink a cupful of the decoction three times a day unless otherwise indicated.

Tinctures

Tinctures comprise the plant in a concentrated liquid form and are taken in small doses. Alcohol is traditionally used in the preparation of tinctures, usually vodka or ethyl alcohol, and this both extracts some of the active principles and preserves the plant. I myself use vegetable glycerol though some glycerols are made from animal by-products. Glycerine is gentle on the stomach and can be tolerated by those who are allergic to regular alcohol. It also tastes slightly sweet and makes the remedies palatable to children without affecting the action of bitters.

Take 50 g (2 oz) of a dried herb and put it in a wide-mouthed jar. Add 150 ml (¼ pint) of boiling water and 250 ml (8 fl oz) of glycerol. Mix together and, if necessary, push the herbs well down so that they are covered by the liquid (or else they will go mouldy). Label the jar and put in a special place for one lunar month, preferably from Full Moon to Full Moon. I leave all my tinctures in my meditation room and let its atmosphere mingle with the plant essences.

Every so often, shake the jar to move the contents around so that they mix evenly. Women who are into witchcraft can do spells and incantations around the tinctures as they brew.

After a month, strain out the liquid and discard the herb – it will make wonderful compost. Put it in a brown or green glass bottle and label it. The tincture should last almost indefinitely; if it does start to go off it will go mouldy. If you make glycerol tinctures in a very hot climate, it is probably best to store them in a fridge as they do not keep so well as those which are alcohol based.

A tincture dosage is 5 to 10 drops taken three times daily before meals, unless otherwise specified. The dose can be taken directly on to the tongue or dropped into water and sipped.

When I am prescribing medicines for other people I usually 'put' a colour into the bottle which I feel is appropriate for that person. To do this I imagine the appropriate colour flooding into the mixture and through the mixture into the person. Visualise a colour such as green or red, and imagine the bottle of medicine being filled with that colour. You can work with colour and herbal remedies by imagining the colour filling the bottle of medicine, so that the essence of the colour mixes with the medicine and is 'taken' with the remedy. Colours can be used in healing; different colours have different qualities. For example, blue is soothing, green healing and red energising.

Fresh herb tinctures

I have recently been experimenting with fresh herb preparations because a fresh plant contains more of the essence of the plant than if it has been dried. This is best done with fleshy plants such as nettle. I do, however, find it rather distressing to put live plants through a liquidizer, so have mixed feelings about this method.

Take a handful of the fresh herb and a small amount of water and put both in a liquidizer or juice extractor. Reduce to a pulp. The amount of water you will need will vary according to the amount of moisture in the plant; add sufficient to keep the blades moving. The resulting liquid should be measured and equal amounts of glycerol added to preserve it. Bottle and label. After a while, the contents will settle and the sediment can be filtered off. This will keep as long as other tinctures but will be thicker and have a characteristic grassy flavour.

Fresh herb tinctures are slightly more dilute and can be taken in larger doses for actue illnesses such as colds and influenza. Dosages up to 1 x 7.5 ml (dessert)spoon are permissable.

Oils and ointments

Herbs lend themselves very well to external application and, with a little enterprise, anyone who can cook can make a herbal oil or ointment. There are many combinations possible, both medicinal and cosmetic. I use the following methods.

Oil

600 ml (1 pint) extra virgin olive oil
50 g (2 oz) dried herb

Mix the ingredients together and let stand in a sunny place for one month. Alternatively, stand the jar in a double boiler and simmer for four hours. Strain.

This oil can be used for massage purposes. I use olive oil because I make large quantities, but if you can afford it, use almond oil. When rubbed on the skin the oil will be absorbed into the blood stream and the herb will act in its usual manner.

Ointment

600 ml (1 pint) herbal oil
3 x 15 ml-4 x 15 ml (3-4 table)spoons lanolin or cocoa butter
50 g (2 oz) beeswax

Gently heat the oil and stir in the lanolin and beeswax. Remove from the heat and beat until cold and thick. The beeswax solidifies the cream and the lanolin emulsifies (makes less greasy), so the proportions can be adjusted accordingly. You can add some tincture to make the cream stronger, about 20 ml (¾ fl oz) to a pint. Most of the creams

I make are fairly greasy, but they do last for quite a long time on the skin.

Essential oils

These are strong preparations. They are oils pressed out of the plants. It is not really possible to do this by yourself, so buy them from herbal suppliers. As they are strong, they should only be used externally, and then only in diluted form. I find them especially useful for inhalations; for example, essential oil of fennel or chamomile for chest infections; or you can use them in the bath for a variety of conditions. Essential oils lend themselves particularly well to treatments of the nervous system and are excellent for insomnia. They can be used for babies and young children whom it would be hard to medicate in any other way. I use about ten to fifteen drops of the oil in the bath or two to five drops in a bowl of water for inhalation. If using essential oils for massage, be sure to dilute them in the ratio of one part essential oil to ten parts almond or olive oil.

WARNING. Never use essential oils directly on the skin as they may burn.

Cough syrups

In the British climate a large number of people suffer from chest complaints, and it is quite useful to know how to make up a cough remedy which will help to clear the chest and not supress a cough. Syrups are essentially herbs preserved in sugar; they are good to sip diluted in hot water.

If I have access to cheap honey, I use this in preference to raw sugar as it has sedative and antiseptic qualities of its own. Honey, however, has water in it so more honey than sugar needs to be added when making the syrup.

50 g (2 oz) dried herbs
1.2 litres (2 pints) cold water
450 g (1 lb) raw brown sugar or
500 g (1¼ lb) honey

Mix together the herbs and water and simmer for thirty minutes. Strain. Return the liquid to the pan and reduce to 600 ml (1 pint). Add the sugar or honey. Stir well until completely dissolved. Pour into clean, warmed bottles. This mixture will last for two to three years.

Dose: 1 x 15 ml (tea)spoonful three or four times daily.

Lotions

A lotion is a water-based substance to be applied externally. Lotions have cooling properties and are best used when a cream would be too greasy or heat-producing, which might aggravate hot conditions such as rashes or inflammations. For a base, I use rosewater, but you could equally use orange flower water or chamomile water. Witch hazel is soothing but quite drying. The flower waters on their own are excellent for burns, rashes, bites and stings, especially sunburn, nappy rash and heat rash because they cool the skin down and stop irritation. I have also used them as a base for mouthwashes and douches to cool inflammations.

The following is an example of how to make a lotion.

Lotion for thrush (oral and vaginal)
100 ml (3½ fl oz) rosewater
5 ml (⅕ fl oz) myrrh
5 ml (⅕ fl oz) tincture of marigold

Mix all ingredients together.

Dose: 1 x 5 ml (tea)spoonful in 300 ml (½ pint) warm water, to be applied to the mouth or vagina as a douche. Use as and when required.

For me, the craft of herbalism has to include the preparation of my own remedies. The yearly seasons and planetary cycles are involved. Witchcraft sees the Goddess as immanent, that is, that She is in everyday things and that the sacred is to be found in the mundane.

I myself have never felt happy about buying bottles of tinctures; I like to be involved in the production process from beginning to end. This means that during the week preceding the Full Moon, I will pick herbs that are ready to be harvested and make up my own tinctures. The process of making a tincture makes me mindful of the Moon and her cycles and I have learned to treat the manufacture of herbal preparation with reverence. It is not just a mundane task to be accomplished. I believe the energy of a herbalist goes into the medicines she makes. If she is rushed or sloppy, her medicines will have the same quality. Whereas if she makes them with love and care, these qualities will mix with the essence of the plant and be taken by the person using the medicine.

I want my patients to have clear, wholesome, powerful medication that is alive and dynamic.

Constituents
This section describes the chemical constituents found in the herbs mentioned in the main text.

Alkaloids
These form the strongest and most varied of all plant constitutents. As their basis many allopathic medicines have naturally occurring plant alkaloids such as morphine, dopamine and mescaline.

Allantoin
Found in the flowering tops of comfrey, allantoin diffuses through the skin to increase the healing time of bones, muscles, ligaments and skin tissue.

Bioflavonoids
Also known as vitamin P, bioflavonoids are found in citrus fruits and some berries (hawthorn). They harden and strengthen blood vessels and have been found to protect against haemorrhage by helping to absorb vitamin C.

Bitters
Bitters are found in many medicinal plants. They work by

reflex; it is the bitter taste which causes the liver and digestive system to respond by increasing its secretions. For this reason liver remedies should not be sweetened to make their taste more palatable. Bitter tonics are used worldwide to help digestion and to act as general cleansing remedies.

Coumarins
Coumarins delay blood clotting by affecting the blood clotting constituents, that is, prothrombin and vitamin K.

Flavones and flavonoid glycosides
These are the most common of plant constituents. They have a variety of actions. They act like bioflavonoids on the circulatory system and are also antispasmodic, diuretic and act as heart stimulants.

Gums and mucilages
These constituents have the common properties of stickiness, they lubricate and cover and protect tissue. Use wherever there is inflammation, to soothe and cool the area, allowing for healing to take place. They are for the lungs, digestive and urinary systems. Mucilages are destroyed by heat, so remedies used for this constituent should be taken cold.

Saponins
Saponins have a structure similar to steroid hormones, and for this reason many plant saponins have been used to form the template for synthetic hormones. The wild yam, for example, formed the basis for the synthesis of sex hormones. Many saponins expel mucus from the lungs. They also aid digestion and absorption, and cleanse and heal the skin.

Tannins
Tannins have an astringent action; they reduce the water content of tissues, bind and reduce secretion and haemorrhage. They are found in many remedies used to heal

wounds and to stop fluxes (expulsions from the body).

Volatile oils
These give plants their particular perfume. Sage, lavender and thyme contain large amounts of volatile oils. These are extracted to make the essential oils used in aromatherapy. Volatile oil is extracted by pouring boiling water over the fresh or dried herb and then covering over with a cloth. Volatile oils have actions in common: they are anti-spasmodic, especially to the gut and lungs, and they are antiseptic, anaesthetic and stimulate digestion. They have a relaxing action on the nervous system.

CONCLUSION

This book is born of a long, winding thread which I took hold of in Amsterdam in 1971 when, as a stranger in a strange land, I was given three books to read by a young man whose name I cannot now recall. One was a book on macrobiotics, the second a herbal, *Back to Eden* and the title of the third eludes me. I read and re-read these books. Through them I discovered the whole world of natural therapeutics. Doors opened and connections were made. Twenty years later, I am still holding that thread and I feel both nearer to its source and yet as far away as ever. Even so, this thread has stayed with me. Here I have spun the thread into a web, connecting the themes of feminism, history, medicine, astrology and women's mysteries. I have rested a while in the centre of the web, wondering at the symmetry and beauty of the different threads. Aware of the delicacy and impermanence of any creation, I hope the winds of change blow the web far and wide and that other spinners will take up the fragments and begin again.

> You may forget but
> Let me tell you
> this: someone in
> some future time
> will think of us

> Sappho.

1 Erasure-'the planned, self serving obliteration throughout

the phallocracy of the lives, words, and achievements of women; the attempted annihilation of the Reality of all others. Example: the attempted obliteration of Sappho's work and reputation. The erasers/obliterators did not fully succeed, however. In Oxyrhyncus, Egypt, between 1897 and 1906, an archeological expedition uncovered papyrus mummy wrappings which had been used to stuff coffins and embalmed animals. In this ancient garbage dump, on wadded strips of papyrus, were the fragmented poems of Sappho.' (From *Websters' First New Intergalactic Wickedary of the English Language*, Conjured by Mary Daly in cahoots with Jane Caputi.)

GLOSSARY OF TERMS

Alteratives: blood cleansers, remedies which act as body purifiers.

Analgesics: pain killing remedies.

Anti-catarrhal remedies: those which reduce phlegm in the body.

Anti-microbial remedies: those which kill pathogenic micro-organisms.

Anti-spasmodic remedies: those which relax muscle spasms in the body.

Astringent remedies: those which dry out the tissues to make them stronger; they stop bleeding and secretions.

Demulcent remedies: those which soothe inflamed tissues.

Diaphoretic remedies: those which induce sweating.

Diuretic remedies: those which increase the production of urine.

Emmenagogic remedies: those which bring on delayed periods.

Expectorant: a remedy which encourages the expulsion of phlegm from the lungs.

Hepatic remedy: for the liver.

Laxative: a remedy to counteract constipation.

Nervine: a remedy for the nervous system.

Sedative: a remedy to relax the nerves.

Soporific: a remedy with a strong sedative action on the nervous system.

Styptic: a remedy to stop the blood flow.

Tonic: an all-round remedy to improve the general level of health.

BIBLIOGRAPHY

Adler, Margot (1979) *Drawing Down the Moon: Witches, Druids, Goddess Worshipers and Other Pagans in America Today*, Beacon Press, Boston.

Appleby, Derek (1985) *Horary Astrology*, Aquarian Books, Wellingborough, Northants.

Assagioli, Roberto (1974) *Psychosynthesis*, Esalen Press, Esalen CA.

Assagioli, Roberto, (1974) *The Act of Will*, Wildwood House, London.

Bailey, Alice, (1982) *Esoteric Astrology*, Lucis Press, London.

Bailey, Alice, (1987) *The Soul and Its Mechanism* Lucis Press, London.

Bairacli de Levy, Juliette, (1974) *The Illustrated Herbal Handbook*, Faber and Faber, London.

Blagrave, (1674) *Supplement to Culpepper's English Physician* William Cole, London.

Boston Womans' Health Book Collective (1984) *Our Bodies, Our Selves*, Simon and Schuster, New York.

British Herbal Medicine Association, Scientific Committee (1976 and 1979) *British Herbal Pharmacopoeia Vols I & II*, British Herbal Medical Association, London.

Brooke, Elisabeth (in press) *A History of Women Healers*.

Buchman, Dian, (1979) *Herbal Medicine*, Rider, London.

Buchman, Dian, (1973) *Feed Your Face*, Duckworth, London.

Budapest Z. (1979) *The Holy Book of Women's Mysteries* Part I, Susan B. Anthony Coven, Oakland, CA.

Budapest Z. (1980), *The Holy Book of Women's Mysteries* Part II, Susan B. Anthony Coven, Oakland, CA.

Cellier, E, (1687) *A Schemme for the Foundation of a Royal Hospital*, London.

Chaff, S., Haimbach, R., Fenichel, C., and Woodside, N. (1977) *Bibliography on Women Physicians* Scarecrow Press, London.

Chancellor, Phillip, (1971) *Handbook of the Bach Flower Remedies*, Daniel, London.

Cirlot, J. E. (1962) *A Dictionary of Symbols*, Routledge & Kegan Paul, London.

Cohn, Norman (1975) *Europe's Inner Demons*, Heineman, London.

Cole, William (1656) *The Art of Simpling*, London.

The Company of Astrologers' Bulletin from the Company of Astrologers, 6 Queens Square, London WC1.

Culpeper, Nicholas (1655) *Culpeper's Astrologicall Judgement of Diseases* William Cole, London.

Culpeper, Nicholas (1655) *Semeiotica Uranica*, William Cole, London.

Culpeper, Nicholas (1656) *Medicaments for the Poor*, William Cole, London.

Culpeper, Nicholas (1654) *A New Method of Physick*, William Cole, London.

Culpeper, Nicholas (1655) *Culpeper's Last Legacy*, William Cole, London.

Culpeper, Nicholas (1659) *Culpeper's School of Physick*, William Cole, London.

Culpeper, Nicholas (1649) *A Physicall Directory*, William Cole, London.

Culpeper, Nicholas (1652) *Galens Art of Physick*, William Cole, London.

Culpeper, Nicholas (1653) *The English Physician, enlarged*, William Cole, London.

Culpeper, Nicholas (1651) *The Emphemeris for 1651*

Cunningham, Donna (1942) *The Astrological Guide to Self Awareness*, CRS Publications, Vancouver.

Daly, Mary (1979) *Gyn/Ecology*, The Women's Press, London.

Davidson, R.C. (1955) *The Technique of Prediction*, Fowler & Co, Essex.

Dworkin, Andrea (1974) *Woman Hating*, Dutton, New York.

Ehrenreich, B. and English, D. (1973) *Witches, Midwives and Nurses*, Feminist Press, New York.

Ferrucci, Piero (1982) *What We May Be*, Turnstone Press, Wellingborough, Northants.

Freeman, Martin (1983) *Forecasting by Astrology*, Aquarian Press, Wellingborough, Northants.

Fulder, Stephen (1980) *The Root of Being*, Hutchinson, London.

Frazer, J.G. (1922) *The Golden Bough*, Macmillan, London.

Gage, Matilda, (1893) *Women Church & State*, second edition, Arno Press, New York 1972.

Gerard, *Herbal* (reprint) (1985) Bracken Books, London.

Gordon, Lesley (1980) *A Country Herbal*, Peerage Books, London.

Gordon, B.L. (1959) *Mediaeval and Renaissance Medicine*, Peter Owen, London.

Graves, Robert (1961) *The White Goddess*, Faber and Faber, London.

Gray, J. (1959) *The Warriors: reflections on men in battle*, New York.

Greene, Liz (1977) *Relating*, Coventure, London.

Greene, Liz (1976) *Saturn*, Aquarian Press, Wellingborough, Northants.

Greene, Liz (1984) *The Astrology of Fate*, George Allen & Unwin, London.

Grieve, M (1931) *A Modern Herbal*, Second edition Peregrine Books, London, (1976).

Griggs, Barbara (1981) *Green Pharmacy*, Jill Norman & Hobhouse, London.

Hand, Robert (1976) *Planets in Transit*, Para Research, Rockport, MA.

Harmer, Juliet (1980) *The Magic of Herbs and Flowers*, Macmillan, London.

Hoffman, David (1983) *The Holistic Herbal* Findhorn Press, Findhorn, Moray, Scotland.

Hoyt, C.A. (1981) *Witchcraft*, South Illinois University Press, Carbondale.

Hughes, M.J. (1943) *Women Healers in Mediaeval Life and Literature*, Kings Crown Press, New York.

Hurd-Mead, K.C. (1938) *A History of Women in Medicine*, Haddam Press, Conneticut, USA.

Hutchins, Alma. R. (1969) *Indian Herbology of North America*, Merco. Ontario, Canada.

Inglis, Brian (1965) *A History of Medicine*, Weidenfeld, London.

Jex-Blake, Dr. Sophia (1886) *Medical Women*, Oliphant, Edinburgh.

Johnson, J. (1657) *The Idea of Practical Physic in Two Books*, trans. N. Culpeper, London.

Jung, Carl Gustav (1964) *Man and His Symbols*, Doubleday & Co, New York.

Kealey, E. (1981) *Mediaeval Medicus*, Johns Hopkins University Press, USA.

Khan, M. Salim (1986) *Islamic Medicine*. Routledge & Kegan Paul, London.

Noriko, Ushida (1968) *Etude comparative de la psychologie d'Aristotle d'avicenne et St Thomas d'Aquin*, Keio Institute of Cultural Studies, Tokyo.

Kieckhefer, R. (1976) *European Witch Trials*, Routledge & Kegan Paul, London and University of California Press, Berkeley.

Kloss, Jethro (1972) *Back to Eden*, Woodbridge, Santa Barbara, CA.

Krutch, Joseph Wood (1976) *Herbal*, Phaidon Press, London.

Langdon-Brown, Sir Walter (1941) *From Witch to Chemotherapy*, Cambridge University Press, Cambridge.

Larner, C. (1981) *Enemies of God – The Witch Hunt in Scotland*, Chatto & Windus, London.

Leland, Charles (1974) *Aradia, Gospel of the Witches*, Samuel Weiser, New York.

Lilly, William (1647) *Christian Astrology*, third edition, 1985 Regulus Publishing, London.

Lilly, William (1651) *Ephemeris 1651*, London.

Lilly, William (1681) *Dr Lilly's last legacy*, London.

Lipinska, M. (1900) *Historic des femmes medicinal*, Librarie G. Jaques & Co, Paris.

Bibliography

Lovejoy, E. (1957) *Women Doctors of the World*, Macmillan, New York.

Lust, John (1974) *The Herb Book*, Bantam Books, New York.

Maclean, I (1980) *The Renaissance Notion of Woman*, Cambridge University Press, Cambridge.

Mariechild, Diane (1981) *Motherwit: A Feminist Guide to Psychic Development*, Crossing Press, New York.

Mayo, Jeff (1980) *Astrology*, Teach Yourself Books.

Mellor, Constance (1975) *Natural Remedies for Common Ailments*, Mayflower, London.

Messegue, Maurice (1979) *Health Secrets of Plants and Herbs*, Collins, London.

Murray, Margaret (1921) *The Witchcult in Western Europe*, Oxford University Press, Oxford.

Neumann, Erich (1955) *The Great Mother*. Bollingen Series, Princetown University press, New Jersey.

Noble, Vicki (1983) *Motherpeace: a way to the goddess through myth, art and tarot*, Harper & Row, San Francisco.

Oaken, Alan (1980) *Complete Astrology*, Bantam Books, London.

Oliver, C.W. (1928) *An analysis of Magic and Witchcraft*, Rider, London.

Owsel, Timkin (1973) *Galen*, Cornell University Press, Cornell.

Packwood, Marlene (1980) *Witchcraft in the Middle Ages*, pamphlet, London.

Palaiseul, Jean (1972) *Grandmother's Secrets*, Penguin, Harmondsworth.

Parvati, Jean (1979) *Hygieia, A Woman's Herbal*, Wildwood House, London.

Perera, Sylvia Brinton (1932) *Descent to the Goddess*, Inner City Books, Toronto, Canada.

Philosophus, William (1651) *Occult Physic*, London.

Plater, F. (1664) *Histories and Observations on Most Diseases Offending the Body*, trans. N. Culpeper, William Cole, London.

Potts, Billie (1981) *Witches Heal, Lesbian Herbal Self Sufficiency*, Hecubas Daughters Inc, New York.

Priest, A.W. and Priest, L.R. (1982) *Herbal Medication*. L.N. Flower, Essex.

Riddle (1985) *Dioscorides on Pharmacy and Medicine*, University of Texas Press.

Riolanus, J. Jnr (1657) *A Sure Guide to Physic and Chyrugery*, London.

River, Lindsay and Gillespie, Sally (1987) *The Knot of Time*, The Women's Press, London.

Riverius, Lazarus (1655) *The Practice of Physic*, trans. N. Culpeper, London.

Rivers, W. H. R. (1924) *Medicine, Magic and Religion*, Kegan Paul, London.

Rohde, E.S. (1922) *Old English Herbals*, Longmans Green & Co, London.

Ruland, M. (1662) *Experimental Physic*, trans. N. Culpeper, London.

Russel, J.B. (1972) *Witchcraft in the Middle Ages*, Cornell University Press, New York.

Sanders, R. (1677) *Student in Physic*, trans. William Lilly, London.

Sasportas, Howard, (1985) *The Twelve Houses*. Aquarian Press, Wellingborough, Northants.

Sibly, E. (1794) *A Key to Physic and Occult Sciences*, London.

Sibly, E. (1794) *The Medical Mirror*, London.

Singer, Dr C. (c. 1920) 'Early English Magic & Medicine', proceedings of the British Academy.

Singer, Dr C. and Underwood, M. (1962) *A Short History of Medicine*, second edition, Clarendon Press, Oxford.

Spretnak, Charlene (1978) *Lost Goddesses of Early Greece*, Moon Books.

Starhawk, (1982) *Dreaming the Dark: Magic, Sex and Politics*, Beacon Press, Boston.

Starhawk, (1989) *The Spiral Dance: A Rebirth of the Ancient Religion of the Great Goddess: Rituals, Invocations, Exercises, Magic*, Harper & Row, San Francisco.

Stone, Merlin (1984) *Ancient Mirrors of Womanhood*, Beacon Press, Boston.

Summers, Rev Montague (1928) *Malleus Maleficarum*, Pushkin Press.

Summers, Rev Montague (1926) *History of Witchcraft and Demonology*, Kegan Paul, London.

Summers, Rev Montague (1927) *The Geography of Witchcraft*, Kegan Paul, London.

Summers, Rev Montague (1928) *The Discovery of Witches*, Cayme Press.

Szaz T. (1971) *The Manufacture of Madness*, Delta Books, London.

Tester, A (1987) *The History of Western Astrology*, Boydell Press, Suffolk.

Thomson, William M.D. (1980) *Healing Plants*, Macmillan, London.

Tindall, G. (1965) *A Handbook on Witches*, Arthur Barker, London.

Trevor-Roper, H.R. (1969) *The European Witch-craze of the 16th & 17th Centuries*, Penguin, London.

Uyldert, Mellie (1980) *The Psychic Garden*, Thorsens, Wellingborough, Northants.

Walker, Barbara (1983) *The Woman's Encyclopedia of Myths and Secrets*, Harper & Row, San Francisco.

Wolkstein, Diane and Kramer, Samuel (1984) *Innana Queen of Heaven and Earth*, Rider, London.

Woodman, Marian (1980) *The Owl Was A Baker's Daughter: Obesity, Anorexia Nervosa and the Repressed Feminine*, Inner City Books, Toronto.

Wren, R.C. (1907) *Potters New Cyclopedia of Botanical Drugs*, Health Science Press, Devon.